Extracorporeal Membrane Oxygenation Support Therapy

Edited by Antonio Loforte

Published in London, United Kingdom

Extracorporeal Membrane Oxygenation Support Therapy
http://dx.doi.org/10.5772/intechopen.101000
Edited by Antonio Loforte

Contributors
Gaik Nersesian, Daniel Lewin, Pia Lanmüller, Sascha Ott, Evgenij Potapov, Tamer Abdalghafoor, Abdulwahid Almulla, Dina Fa Alwaheidi, Ali Kindawi, Amr Salah Omar, Maria M. Crespo, Christian A. Bermudez, Pilje Kang, Ahmed Said, Neel Shah, Andrea Lechiancole, Igor Vendramin, Sandro Sponga, Ugolino Livi, Massimo Maiani, Aggeliki Gkouziouta, Sunit Singla, Ashley K. Binder, Gabriella Rovero, Ciara Hanley, Cathal MacDonncha, Rachel Jooste, John Laffey, Antonio Loforte, Gregorio Gliozzi, Giulio Giovanni Cavalli, Carlo Mariani, Luca Botta, Nazzareno Galiè, Davide Pacini, Sofia Martin-Suarez

First published in London, United Kingdom, 2023 by IntechOpen
IntechOpen is the global imprint of INTECHOPEN LIMITED, registered in England and Wales, registration number: 11086078, 5 Princes Gate Court, London, SW7 2QJ, United Kingdom

British Library Cataloguing-in-Publication Data
A catalogue record for this book is available from the British Library

Additional hard and PDF copies can be obtained from orders@intechopen.com

Extracorporeal Membrane Oxygenation Support Therapy
Edited by Antonio Loforte
p. cm.
Print ISBN 978-1-80356-548-4
Online ISBN 978-1-80356-549-1
eBook (PDF) ISBN 978-1-80356-550-7

Meet the editor

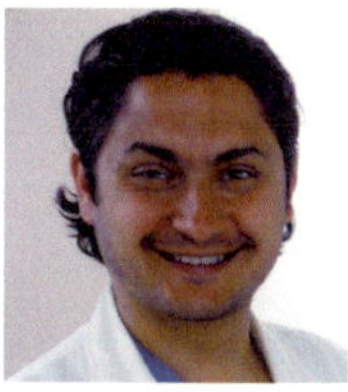

Dr. Antonio Loforte, MD, Ph.D., is a senior staff surgeon and chair of the Mechanical Circulatory Support (MCS) Program at the Department of Surgical Sciences, University of Turin, and the City of Health and Science Hospital Turin, University Division of Cardiac Surgery, Heart and Lung Transplant Center, Italy. He completed his cardiothoracic surgery training at the University of Bologna, S. Orsola University Hospital, IRCCS Bologna, Italy; S. Camillo-Forlanini Hospital, Rome, Italy; St. Antonius Ziekenhuis, Nieuwegein, the Netherlands; and the Deutsches Herzzentrum Berlin, Germany. He additionally joined the Michael E. DeBakey Department of Surgery, Division of Transplant and Assist Devices, Houston, Texas, USA. Dr. Loforte is an active member of several professional organizations including the European Association for Cardio-Thoracic Surgery (EACTS), Society of Thoracic Surgeons (STS), International Society for Heart and Lung Transplantation (ISHLT), American Society for Artificial Internal Organs (ASAIO), International Society for Mechanical Circulatory Support (ISMCS), Roland Hetzer International Cardiothoracic and Vascular Surgery Society (RHICS), Extracorporeal Life Support Organization (ELSO), European Society for Organ Transplantation (ESOT), Società Italiana di Chirurgia Cardiaca (SICCH), and Società Italiana dei Trapianti d'Organo e di Tessuti (SITO), among others. His scientific research focuses mostly on heart transplantation and MCS issues. He serves as a reviewer for several international journals and is an editorial board member for 10 of them. He is the associate editor for the 'Implantable MCS Section' of *Artificial Organs*. He belongs to the ISHLT Standard and Guidelines Committee, ISHLT Cardiogenic Task Force, and ISHLT MCS Operative Committee (co-chair). He received a 'European Ph.D.' label in Organ Transplantation and several international awards in Europe and the United States. Recently, Dr. Loforte was appointed president-elect of ISMCS and Professor of Cardiac Surgery at the University of Turin, Italy.

Contents

Preface

Extracorporeal membrane oxygenation (ECMO), also known as extracorporeal life support (ECLS), has evolved from a salvage form of life support, used only in cases in which all other therapies have failed, to a mainstream therapy for patients experiencing acute cardiac and/or respiratory failure. Initial experiences were associated with poor outcomes and few survivors. Challenges to success included difficulties in optimal patient selection, crudely designed and implemented technologies, an unclear understanding of the relationship between the patient and the extracorporeal circuit, lack of management guidelines, and difficulties in managing complications and guiding patients. However, over the past 20–30 years, there has been a growing recognition of the potentially life-saving benefits of the role of extracorporeal support in allowing the failing heart/lungs to heal, possibly allowing for recovery or serving as a bridge to more definitive end-organ replacement therapy such as ventricular assist devices or transplantation. This evolution has reflected a long journey, one that continues to evolve in part due to the hard work, dedication, and overall commitment of those who recognize the tremendous potential of ECMO to bring hope and restore life to those who would otherwise die.

ECMO is a rapidly evolving and extremely complex technology. With a better understanding of the technology, the indications for support, patient selection, surgical approach, and ECMO management, the outcomes will continue to improve.

Developing a comprehensive "ECMO team" is the first step in building a successful program. This team must be prepared to initiate therapy at any time and in any setting, from those as controlled as an operating room to those as chaotic as an emergency room. While the specific members of the team might vary from program to program, there are several key features that must be established in advance. It is well recognized that effective teams must communicate and work well together. There must be uniform trust and a collective value attached to the expertise that each member brings to the bedside. Additionally, there must be a willingness to embrace the concepts of crew resource management (CRM). The foundation of CRM is that every member of the team has a voice and that each voice is valued and respected. All members of the team must be encouraged, if not empowered, to speak up, particularly when there are safety concerns. In the context of an ECMO team, membership must include all ECMO-related disciplines.

This book discusses general clinical topics related to the specifics of therapy. There are chapters on cardiogenic shock, severe acute respiratory distress syndrome, and generalized applications for longer-term support. The book also addresses the fundamental differences between veno-veno ECMO (VV-ECMO) for pulmonary support and veno-arterial ECMO (VA-ECMO) for cardiac or cardiopulmonary support. This book reflects the collective teamwork of those individuals worldwide who have dedicated countless energy to achieving a better understanding of those ECMO details that will ultimately yield better outcomes.

Dr. Antonio Loforte, MD, Ph.D.,
Chair,
Mechanical Circulatory Support (MCS) Program,
Department of Surgical Sciences,
University of Turin,
Turin, Italy

City of Health and Sciences Hospital Turin,
University Division of Cardiac Surgery,
Heart and Lung Transplant Center,
Turin, Italy

Chapter 1

ECMO in Cath-Lab for Coronary, Structural or Combined Percutaneous Cardiac Interventional High-Risk Procedure

Gabriella Rovero

Abstract

This chapter describes the use of ECMO for interventional cardiology procedures. In recent years, the rapid development of these techniques has allowed treatment of extremely complex patients, not subject to traditional cardiac surgery due to the very high operational risk which was, therefore, intended only for palliative medical therapy. These procedures are carried out by a multidisciplinary team composed of an interventional cardiologist, heart surgeon, anaesthetist, and perfusionist who collaborate closely during all phases of the patient's hospitalisation.

Keywords: ECMO, complex intervention, heart failure, invasive cardiac support, TAVI

1. Introduction

Veno-arterial extracorporeal membrane oxygenation (V-A ECMO) is a temporary, mechanical, circulatory, and respiratory support system. Its main use is in patients with heart and/or respiratory failure, allowing complete support by ensuring continuous systemic perfusion and oxygenation.

This support system has traditionally been used as "rescue" therapy in patients with cardiogenic shock. However, ECMO implantation in emergency conditions is burdened by relevant mortality and morbidity, due to high vascular complications and reduced coronary reserve of patients with severe aortic stenosis or complex coronary artery disease, especially in the presence of a reduction of the global systolic function. In these cases, prolonged hypotension can lead to a rapid deterioration of hemodynamic conditions with the development of cardio-metabolic shock.

Recently, the use of ECMO as support during percutaneous complex cardiac interventions has been proposed, especially in high-risk patients. Besides the clinical aspects, also some technical issues have to be taken into account, such as complex anatomies with an extensive ischemic area at risk and severe impaired ventricular systolic function.

2. Indications

Interventional cardiology procedures, both for valvular and coronary diseases, have become increasingly complex in recent years. Patients to be treated often have multiple comorbidities that make cardiac surgery impractical because it is of very high risk. The development of new technologies has made it possible to treat patients who, until a few years ago, were destined only for palliative medical therapy. The need to treat these patients considered inoperable, he pushed the haemodynamist to use an "extracorporeal circulation" also in the haemodynamic room, in order to carry out very complex procedures both from a clinical and technical point of view in "safety." The literature shows how ECMO or in any case an extracorporeal circulation installed in an emergency regime is burdened by very high mortality and morbidity, especially in patients who have a reduced cardiac and respiratory reserve, where prolonged hypotension can rapidly evolve towards cardio-metabolic shock [1–4]. Veno-arterial extracorporeal membrane oxygenation (ECMO), therefore, initially conceived as a rescue therapy in emergencies and cardiogenic shock has become a "protection" tool for patients and operators [5–9]. The procedures that can be performed with the aid of extracorporeal assistance are many and can be performed individually or combined with each other, including TAVI [10–14], mitral valve [15–17] or percutaneous tricuspid repair, percutaneous coronary intervention [18–23], and electrophysiology procedures, such as ablations of ventricular tachycardias [24–26].

2.1 Main indications for the prophylactic use of ECMO

- Reduced left ventricular ejection fraction. It represents the most common indication. Patients with depressed ventricular function and aortic stenosis, whether or not it is associated with coronary heart disease to be submitted to TAVI, they may, during the stages of the procedure, not tolerate the hypotensive phase resulting, for example, from rapid ventricular stimulation during the release of the prosthesis. And as shown by the literature, the installation of ECMO in an emergency is burdened with a high mortality and high complication rate [10–13].

- Severe aortic valve stenosis associated with coronary artery disease involving the left main, treatable with concomitant TAVI and angioplasty. Angioplasty performed on the left main (performed before valvular treatment) could lead, even in this case, to severe hypotension or potentially fatal arrhythmias in a patient with concomitant severe aortic stenosis, even more so if with depressed systolic function.

- Severe coronary artery disease (usually involving the left main or equivalent) in patients with severe chronic respiratory failure, even with normal left ventricular function. Based on our experience, it was necessary to treat a patient in work-up for inclusion in the lung transplant list for severe and extensive pulmonary fibro¬sis after COVID-19 pneumonia, suffering from a 90% stenosis of the distal left main coronary artery, involving the ostia of the anterior descending artery and circumflex and had an intermediate branch of large calibre and distribution occluded, in a left-dominated coronary circle. Patients like this (not subject to coronary artery bypass surgery both due to the need for mechanical ventilation for cardiac surgery with probable weaning difficulties and increased infectious risk, and due to the risk of damage to grafts in subsequent bipulmonary transplant surgery) are exposed to a very high risk of acute respiratory failure with minimal cardiac defiance during the revascularization procedure. Other left ventricular assistance systems, such as the Impella (axial pump, without the possibility of adding an oxygenator), are, therefore, not sufficient to guarantee that the procedure will be safely carried out, unlike ECMO, which allows the patient to be kept alert, spontaneously breathing with stable hemodynamic.

- Combined valve disorders in patients with severe left ventricular impairment, for example, severe aortic valve stenosis or insufficiency to undergo TAVI and severe mitral insufficiency to undergo Mitraclip (Abbott) in the same session. The use of the ECMO in these cases allows the interventional procedure to be assimilated into real heart surgery.

- Severe coronary artery disease ("high-risk PCI") in patients who cannot receive other assistance systems, such as Impella (Abiomed, Danvers, MA, USA), due to the presence of a mechanical aortic valve prosthesis.

- In some cases, in addition to the prophylactic action aimed at hemodynamic stability during the procedure, the assistance can also be used to facilitate the technical development of the procedure. In patients, for example, with severe or massive tricuspid regurgitation and severe depression of the right ventricular function, subjected to percutaneous repair of the tricuspid valve with the "edge-to-edge" technique (i.e., Triclip, Abbott), the venous drainage guaranteed by the ECMO allows the reduction of diameters of the right ventricle and the consequent reduction of the coaptation gap between the tricuspid flaps, thus favouring the implantation of the clips. The conduction of assistance in these cases must be very accurate to avoid the return to an initial right ventricular volume, causing a laceration of the tricuspid flaps or the detachment of the positioned clips, therefore continuous transoesophageal control is essential.

3. Pre-procedural phase

A "Heart Team" made up of interventional cardiologists, cardiac surgeons, clinical cardiologists, cardio anesthesiologists and perfusionists discusses the clinical characteristics of all patients. The traditional cardiac surgery option is excluded due to the high operative risk (Euroscore II, STS score, and Syntax score), and the percutaneous option is chosen for the treatment of the diseases in question. But even these procedures are not free from risks, and in certain situations (clinical or technical), it is necessary to carry them out using mechanical assistance to the circulation. Several factors push the Heart Team to perform coronary or percutaneous valve procedures in ECMO assistance, [27] including acute heart failure, hemodynamic instability, reduced ejection fraction, need for support with inotropic drugs, extremely high surgical risk, technical aspects, particularly, for complex myocardial revascularizations with large areas of myocardial risk and risk of haemodynamic destabilisation during the procedure. Hemodynamic instability is defined as the need for inotropic drugs to maintain an average arterial pressure > 65 mmHg, while electrical instability refers to the presence of relapses of ventricular arrhythmias sustained in the last 24 hours.

In addition to routine instrumental and laboratory tests (ECG, chest x-ray, blood chemistry with control of blood counts, renal and hepatic function, and a particular focus on coagulation screening), a transthoracic or transoesophageal echocardiogram is performed if required by the underlying pathology. All patients are then subjected to an aortic CT angiography, which allows to evaluate the course, calibres, presence, and extent of atheromasia/calcifications or other alterations (e.g., aneurysms and thrombotic apposition) along the entire arterial tree and, therefore, allows to choose which is the best site for the assistance installation.

In some patients, especially those who are suffering from valvular pathologies with reduced ejection fraction and/or pulmonary hypertension, the infusion of Levosimendan in the 24–48 hours preceding the procedure may be useful in order to make them arrive at the best possible compensation conditions for the procedure. This may favour the weaning of the patient from extracorporeal circulation and limit or in any case reduce the need for the use of inotropic drugs in the intra- or post-procedural period.

4. Circuit and cannulation techniques

The standard configuration for interventional cardiology procedures is a peripheral veno-arterial extracorporeal membrane oxygenation (V-A ECMO), with cannulation of the femoral artery and vein. They are usually using high-flow arterial cannulas (18-20Fr) and multistage venous cannulas with the distal end positioned in the superior vena cava under fluoroscopic guidance (**Figures 1–3**).

Cannulation can be performed under echography guidance, with percutaneous technique (with the use of percutaneous devices of haemostasis, such as Proglide (Abbott Park, IL, USA) or Manta (Teleflex, USA)) or with surgical isolation of the femoral vessels, depending on the anatomical characteristics of the patient. Based on the pre-procedural CT analysis, arterial cannulation sites other than the femoral arteries can be chosen, when these are not suitable for use due to insufficient calibres or extreme atheroma (**Figures 4–6**).

The most frequently used alternative site is the axillary artery, which, in most cases, has an adequate calibre to ensure systemic perfusion with the advantage of offering an antegrade flow and is rarely affected by atheromatous or calcific processes.

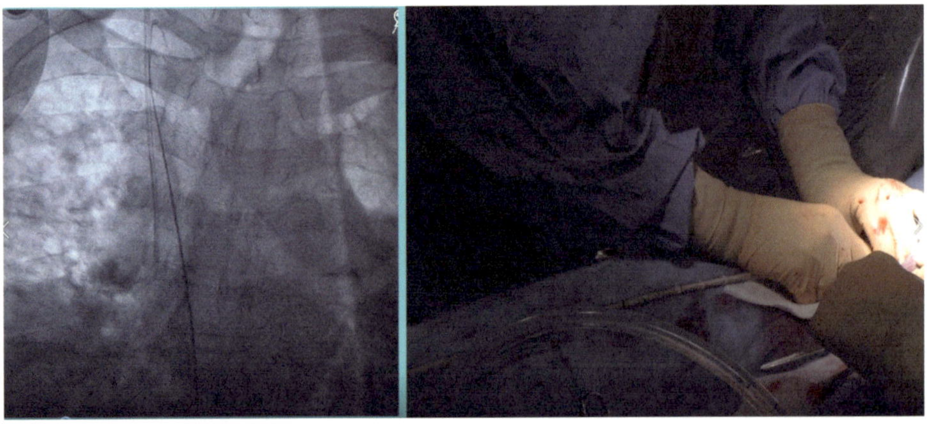

Figure 1.
Placement of the venous cannula in the superior vena cava.

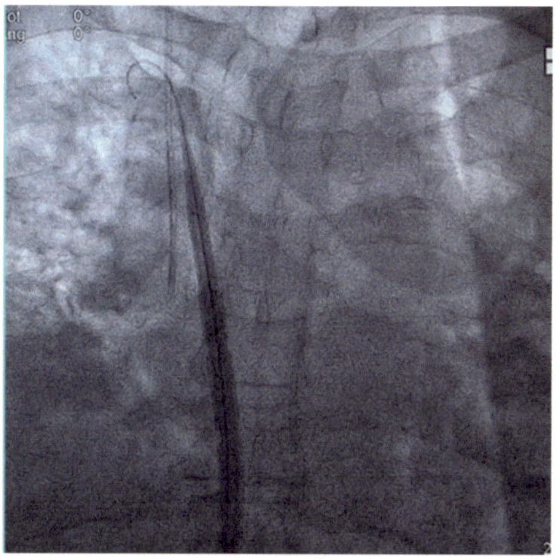

Figure 2.
Control of venous cannula positioning.

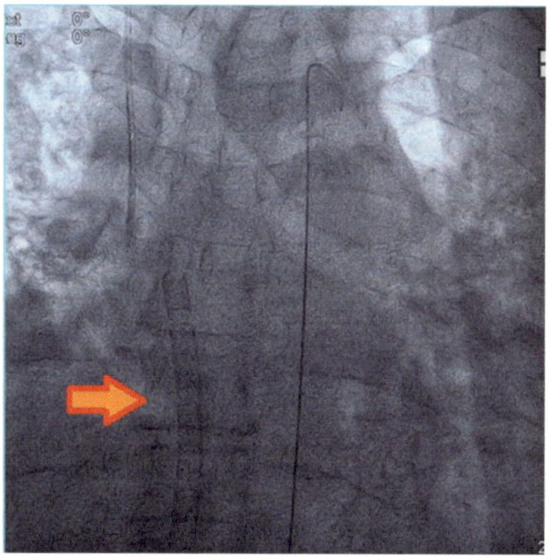

Figure 3.
Venous cannula in superior vena cava.

The standard circuit, consisting of venous and arterial lines connected to a centrifugal pump, oxygenator, and heat exchanger, can be processed according to the needs deriving from the patient's pathology or technical characteristics of the procedure. For example, it may be necessary to unload the left ventricle (i.e., TAVI procedures in cases of severe aortic regurgitation), which is carried out with the introduction of catheters of adequate calibre in the left ventricle (not less than 6 Fr) inserted with transseptal or transaortic approach or in the pulmonary artery through the femoral or jugular vein and connected on the venous line (**Figures** 7 and **8**).

The use of a percutaneous left ventricular drainage that limits ventricular distension, in cases of severe aortic regurgitation [28], guarantees greater procedural hemodynamic stability and facilitates the release of the aortic valve prosthesis for the correction of the regurgitation itself (in fact, it allows to obtain the almost total absence of systolicization of the left ventricle, a function similar to rapid ventricular

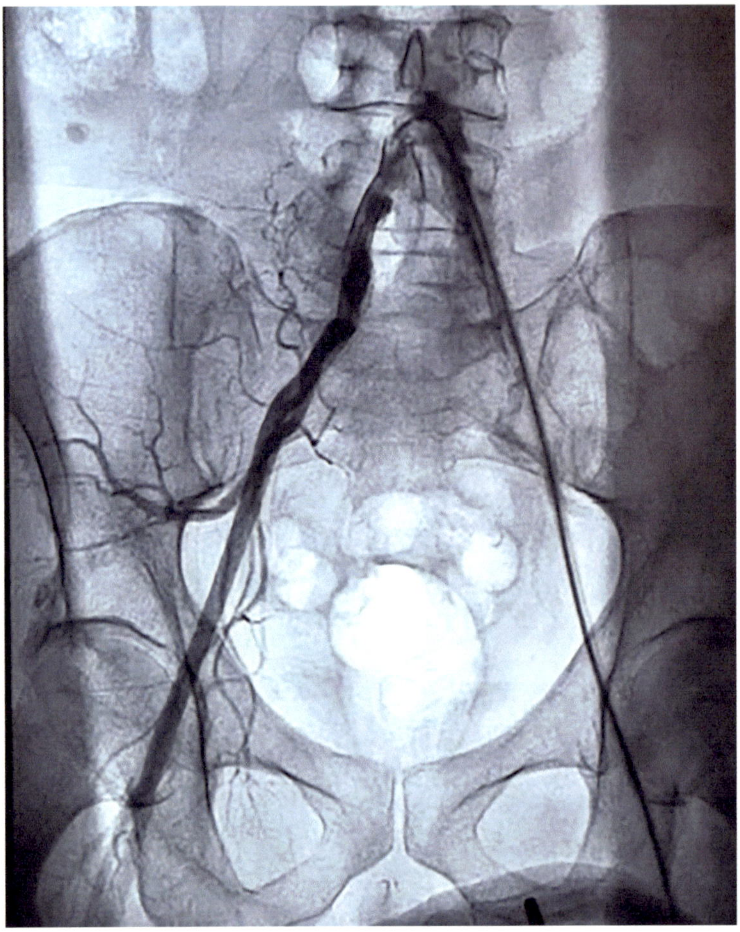

Figure 4.
Angiographic control prior to arterial puncture at the site chosen for cannulation, performed from the contralateral arterial access.

stimulation, limiting the risk of "pop up" of the valve prosthesis). Limiting ventricular distension and the consequent increase in oxygen consumption is a crucial factor in limiting the hemodynamic and arrhythmic instability of a heart in critical conditions and can, therefore, represent strength in the treatment of situations, such as cardiogenic shock or the complications of percutaneous interventions. In fact, the ECMO protects the entire organism from the low cardiac output deriving from a condition of cardiogenic shock, but paradoxically the least protected organ is the heart itself because it undergoes distension of its cavities with an increase in oxygen requirements (Law of Laplace) and, therefore, the risk of ischemia. The possibility of draining the left cavities reduces this problem and makes the manoeuvres to remedy any complications more effectively (i.e., defibrillation in case of serious arrhythmias or repositioning of an aortic prosthesis for massive regurgitation).

In other cases, double venous cannulation, both femoral and jugular, may be necessary, for example for the treatment of tricuspid regurgitation, where the encumbrance of the single multistage cannula in the right atrium (diameter 22–23 Fr) would not allow the passage of catheters (with a diameter of 24Fr in the case of the Triclip) and the manoeuvres of percutaneous tricuspid repair. In these cases, a cannula is

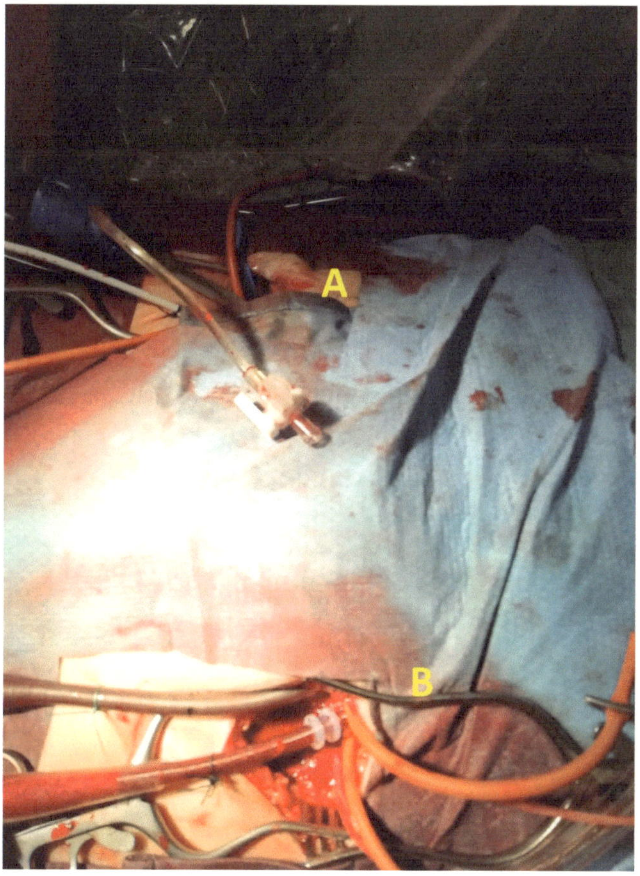

Figure 5.
Surgical femoral accesses for TAVI (A) and ECMO (B).

placed in the inferior vena cava with the upper end at the level of the hepatic veins and a second cannula in the right internal jugular vein (14–17Fr) is added, with the end at the level of the superior atrio-caval junction for ensuring adequate venous drainage (**Figures 9–11**).

In addition, leads can be created on the arterial line to allow procedures to be performed with a single arterial access (especially PCI or in TAVI procedures for the passage of the reference pigtail for valve implantation), obviously, in these cases, it must be carried out a careful evaluation of the resistance to flow deriving from the encumbrance provided by the catheter inside the arterial line, so that sufficient systemic perfusion is guaranteed without increasing the risk of haemolysis, which would nullify the advantage of "saving" arterial access to the patient.

5. Procedural phase—conduct of assistance

Most patients do not require intubation and mechanical ventilation, so the procedures can be performed with the patient in spontaneous breathing, mildly sedated, especially for analgesic purposes, by practising local anaesthesia at the site of the vascular accesses. In some cases, the interventional procedure to be performed

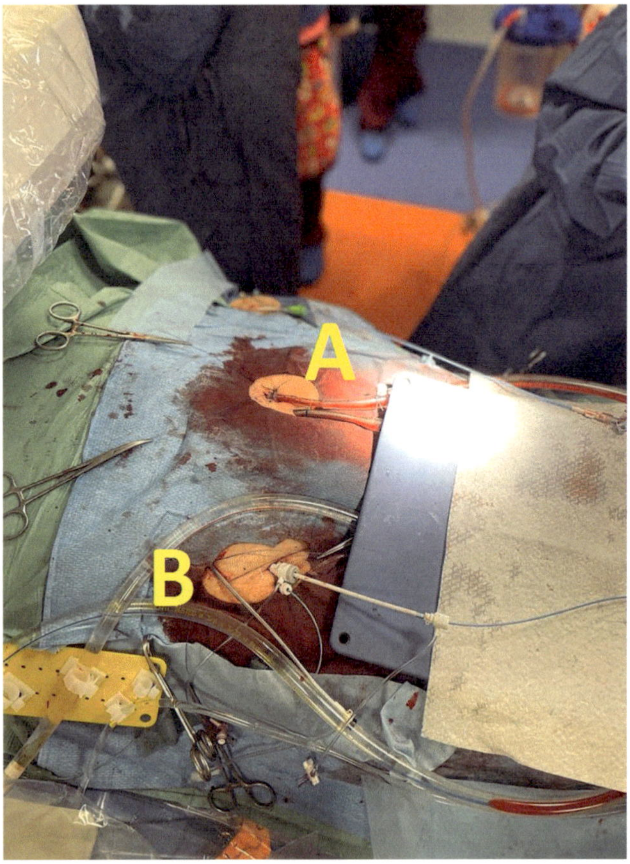

Figure 6.
Percutaneous femoral accesses for ECMO (A) and coronary angioplasty (B).

requires continuous transoesophageal monitoring (i.e., Mitraclip), in these cases, it is preferable to practice general anaesthesia and mechanically ventilate the patient. In the case of intubation, lung-protective ventilation is performed during extracorporeal assistance and the gas supplied to the oxygenator is adjusted to achieve an arterial oxygen partial pressure of approximately 150 mmHg and normocapnia.

In all cases, the blood pressure is monitored and a central venous catheter is positioned for the measurement of the central venous pressure and the possible rapid administration of liquids or drugs. In addition, a bladder catheter is placed for monitoring diuresis.

Vascular access is performed under ultrasound guidance for the positioning of the small calibre introducers (usually 7-8Fr) necessary for both the positioning of the cannula for ECMO and for the execution of the interventional procedure. Once inserted, systemic heparinization is carried out, administering a quantity of heparin necessary to achieve an ACT (activating clotting time) of 250 sec (about 200 IU/kg). Once this value has been reached, the arterial and venous cannulas are positioned and extracorporeal circulation is started, usually in normothermia.

In most cases, total replacement of the pump and respiratory function is not required, but assistance is provided to the circulation, maintaining a flow equal to

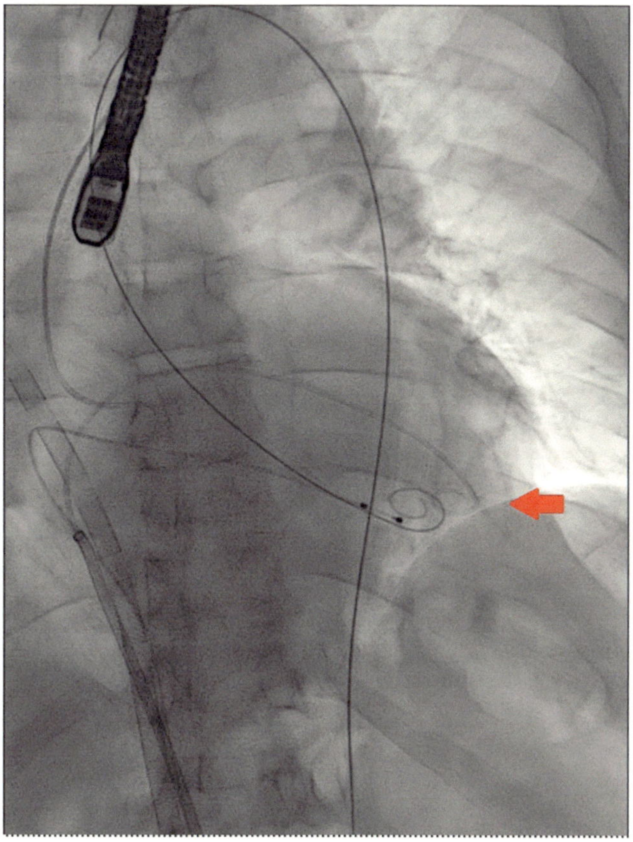

Figure 7.
The arrow indicates transseptal pigtails for unloading the left ventricle during the TAVI procedure for severe aortic regurgitation.

approximately 70% of the total theoretical flow, and calculated on the basis of the patient's body surface. During the various phases of the procedure, the flow will be modified according to the specific needs of the procedure itself, for example, it is reduced to a minimum during the release of the aortic prostheses in order to avoid a "pop down" of the prosthesis itself inside the left ventricle conversely, during manoeuvres, such as coronary rotational atherectomy, the flow is increased in order to support the circulation and facilitate the washing of intracoronary debris. As happens in cardiac surgery operating rooms, close and continuous collaboration between the operators and the perfusionist is, therefore, essential.

Every 30 minutes of extracorporeal assistance, a blood gas examination and ACT check are performed to monitor the patient's respiratory exchanges and metabolic balance.

At the end of the procedure, the pump flow is gradually weaned. If necessary, inotropic drugs can be used to promote hemodynamic stability. This operation can take from a few tens of minutes to a few hours, depending on the patient's needs. In case of impossibility of weaning (which has never happened in our experience), the ECMO can be kept at adequate flow, transferring the patient to the intensive care unit where slow weaning will be attempted in the following days.

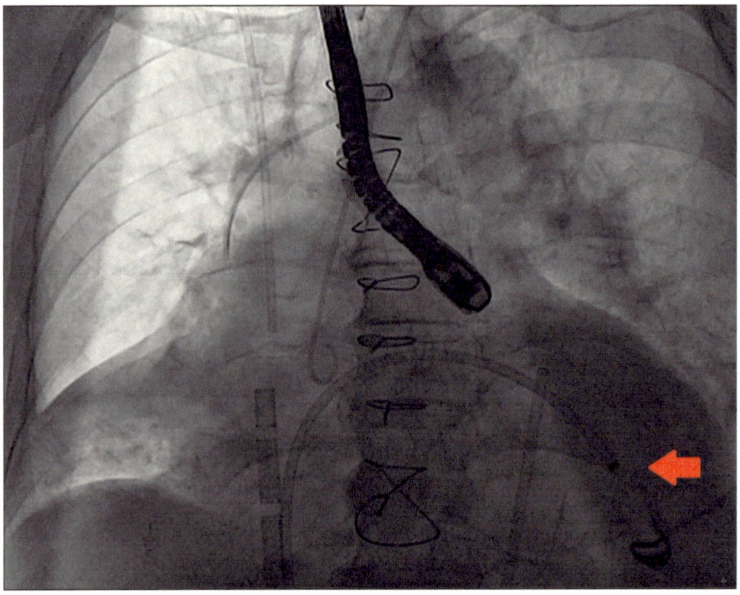

Figure 8.
The arrow indicates 8Fr catheter for unloading the left ventricle inserted transseptally during a combined procedure of TAVI and Mitraclip in a patient with severe aortic and mitral regurgitation.

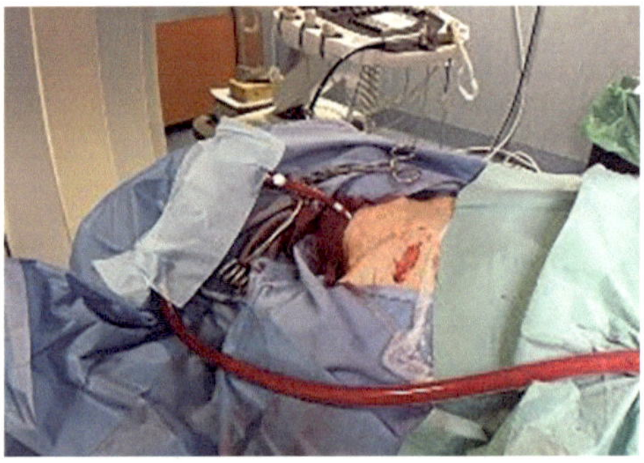

Figure 9.
Cannula positioned in the right internal jugular vein and connected to the venous line.

Upon obtaining stable and valid hemodynamic at the complete weaning of care, the cannula can be removed and the protamine sulphate is administered.

In cases of surgical isolation, decannulation will be directed with surgical repair of the vessels (usually with the closure of previously packaged purse-string suture). In cases of percutaneous implantation, arterial decannulation is performed, when possible, by placing and inflating at low atmospheres, a haemostasis balloon of adequate calibre (usually at least 2 mm greater than the diameter of the external iliac artery) upstream from the cannulation site, by crossover of the femoral arteries or through a guide inserted in the radial artery and pushed up to the affected femoral, which allows the removal of the cannula itself and the closure of the femoral breach with the means of percutaneous haemostasis

DOI: http://dx.doi.org/10.5772/intechopen.105933

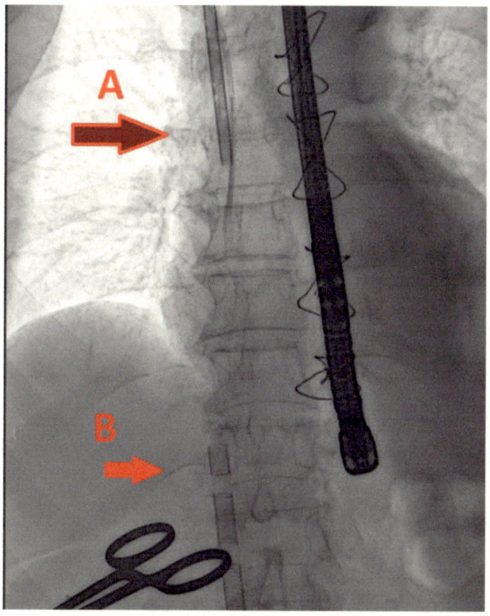

Figure 10.
Cannula in superior vena cava (A) and inferior vena cava with the tip at the level of the hepatic veins (B).

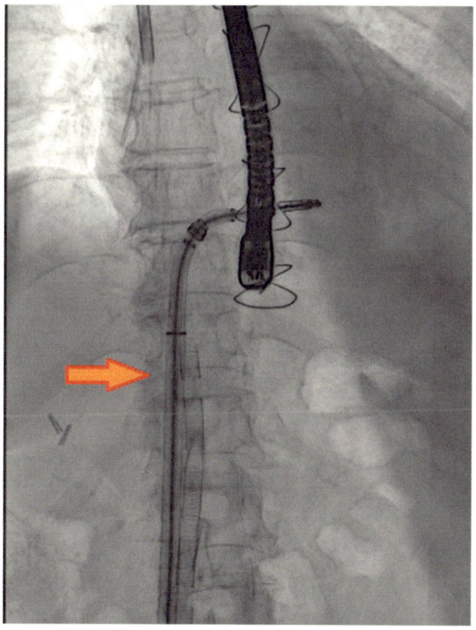

Figure 11.
Percutaneous repair procedure of the tricuspid valve with the Triclip system—the arrow indicates the final position of the venous cannula at the level of the hepatic veins to allow manoeuvres for the delivery of the Triclip in the right atrium.

(Proglide or Manta) by limiting blood losses as much as possible (**Figures 12–15**). As for percutaneous venous decannulation, an external suture can be applied or a Proglide can be used.

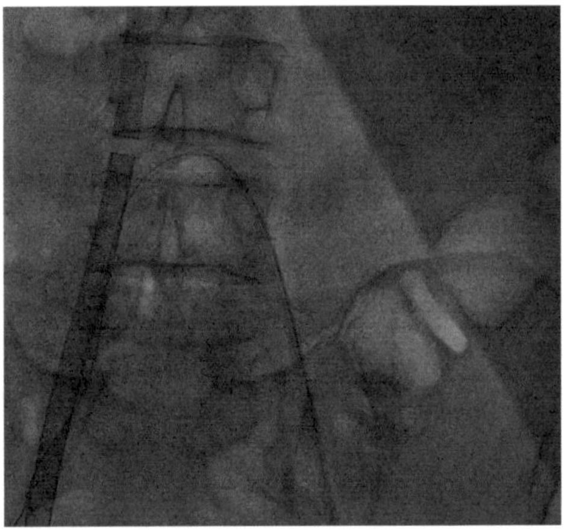

Figure 12.
Femoral artery crossover.

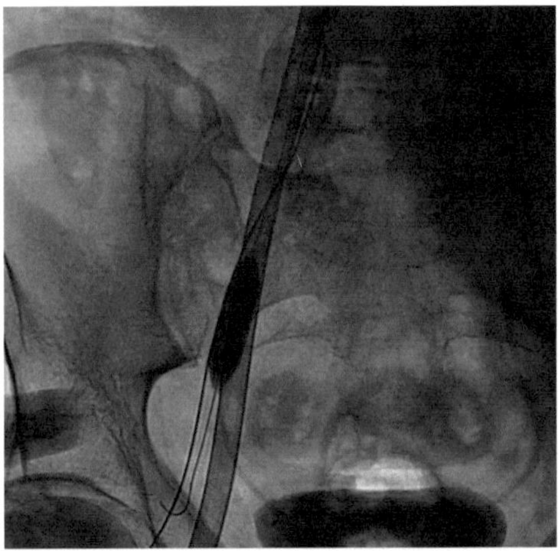

Figure 13.
Haemostasis balloon placed in the right iliac artery for removal of the arterial introducer at the end of a TAVI procedure.

Once haemostasis is achieved, compression dressings are applied to the access sites and the patient is transferred to the intensive care unit for monitoring for the first 24 hours.

6. Conclusion

Our experience in the prophylactic use of ECMO in Cath-lab for the treatment of extremely complex patients has shown good results in both the short- and medium-term. The success of this therapeutic strategy was confirmed by the medium-term results, considering that most of these patients, due to their age and basic clinical conditions, would have been destined for palliative medical therapy and a certain poor short-term prognosis [21–29].

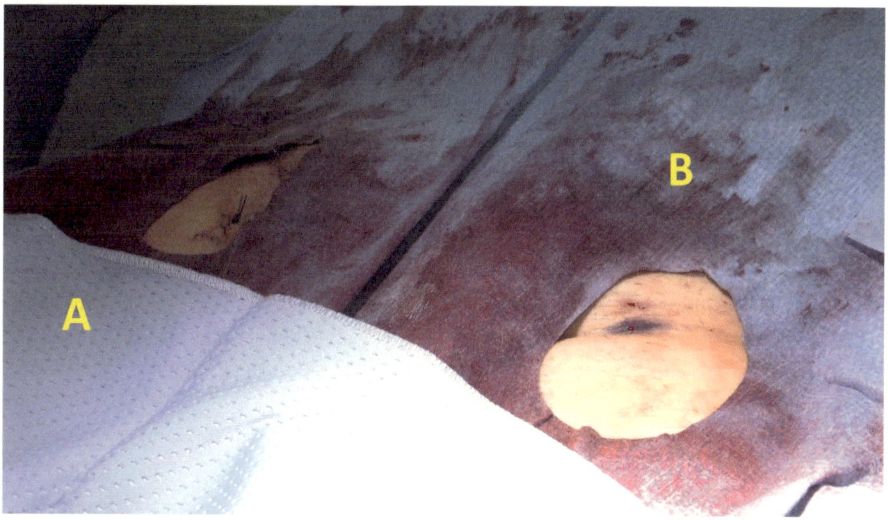

Figure 14.
Outcome of ECMO percutaneous femoral access (A) and coronary angioplasty (B).

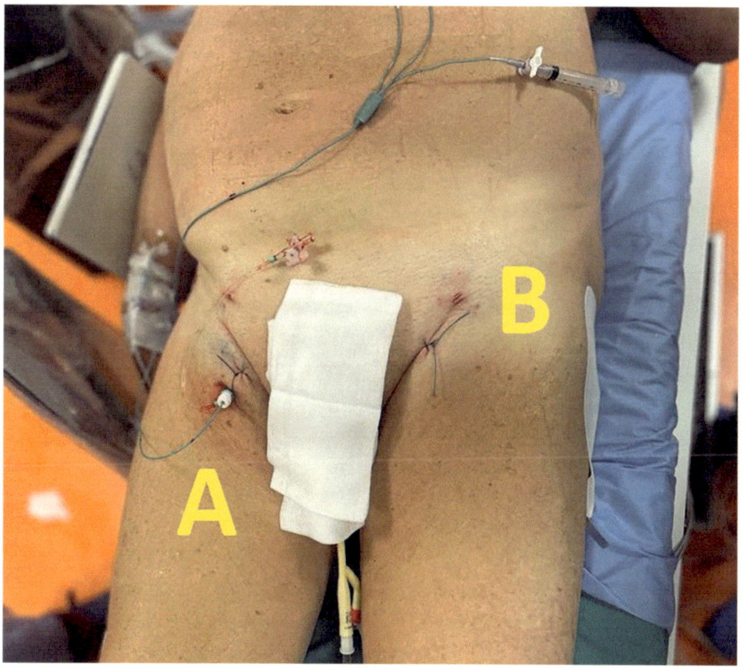

Figure 15.
TAVI (A) and ECMO (B) percutaneous femoral access outcome.

V-A ECMO was mainly used in the "bail-out" to address conditions of severe respiratory distress or refractory cardiogenic shock. Recently, however, its prophylactic use in the interventional cardiology laboratory has been considered, especially in complex and high-risk coronary procedures, showing good results and to a lesser extent for structural interventional procedures (TAVI) with good results in terms of procedural "security."

Although there are no standardised criteria for defining a "high-risk" procedure, there is general consensus due to a variable combination of clinical and anatomical factors. Among the first are the presence of a compromised functional class (NYHA III/IV), ventricular dysfunction, pulmonary hypertension, haemodynamic or electrical instability, heart failure despite optimised therapy, and the presence of comorbidities. Among the latter include the extent and anatomy of coronary lesions, the extent of the ischemic area at risk during the procedure, the need to use "aggressive" devices (i.e. rotational atherectomy) and anatomical features of the valves. Furthermore, the clinical criticality of the patient may be due to the coexistence of coronary and valvular or plurivalvular disease requiring combined treatment causing an inexorable increase in procedural risk.

The presence of a multidisciplinary team expert in the treatment of complex diseases, which collaborates in the management of the entire length of hospitalisation of these patients is, therefore, fundamental. Starting from the correct choice of the procedure for each individual patient, to the planning of each step of the procedure itself and the intra- and post-procedural management with the active and productive comparison of each specialist.

Further studies are obviously needed to confirm the good results of the currently limited experiences, but we are confident that the use of ECMO to carry out this type of procedure represents an important therapeutic option in the near future.

Acknowledgements

Thanks to the entire medical and nursing team of Maria Pia Hospital in Turin, which allowed us to perform these complex and innovative procedures. A special thanks to Dr. Elvis Brscic and Dr. Katiuscia Testa who with so much passion, courage, a pinch of madness, and above all a lot of hard work have allowed the realisation of the "ECMO in Cath-lab" project.

Conflict of interest

The author declares no conflict of interest.

Author details

Gabriella Rovero
Maria Pia Hospital, GVM Care and Research, Turin, Italy

*Address all correspondence to: gabriella.rovero@gmail.com

References

[1] Khorsandi M, Dougherty S, Bouamra O, et al. Extracorporeal membrane oxygenation for refractory cardiogenic shock after adult cardiac surgery: A systematic review and meta-analysis. Journal of Cardiothoracic Surgery. 2017;**12**:55

[2] Oliver H, Andreas H, Alois P, Julio N, Vicente B, Thomas M, et al. Emergency and prophylactic use of miniaturized veno-arterial extracorporeal membrane oxygenation in transcatheter aortic valve implantation. Catheterization and Cardiovascular Interventions. 2013;**82**:E542-E551

[3] Raffa GM, Kowalewski M, Meani P, Follis F, Martucci G, Arcadipane A, et al. ECMO in TAVI investigators Group (ETIG). In-hospital outcomes after emergency or prophylactic veno-arterial extracorporeal membrane oxygenation during transcatheter aortic valve implantation: A comprehensive review of the literature. Perfusion. 2019;**34**(5):354-363. DOI: 10.1177/0267659118816555

[4] Burzotta F, Russo G, Basile E, Aurigemma C, Leone AM, Niccoli G, et al. Come orientarsi tra contropulsatore, Impella e ossigenazione a membrana extracorporea. Giornale Italiano di Cardiologia. 2018;**19** (6 Suppl.):5S-13S

[5] Guerrero-Miranda Cesar Y, Hall SA. Cardiac catheterization and percutaneous intervention procedures on extracorporeal membrane oxygenation support. Annals of Cardiothoracic Surgery. 2019;**8**(1):123-128

[6] Rihal CS, Naidu SS, Givertz MM, et al. 2015 SCAI/ACC/HFSA/STS clinical expert consensus statement on the use of percutaneous mechanical circulatory support devices in cardiovascular care (endorsed by the American Heart Association, the Cardiological Society of India, and Sociedad Latino Americana de Cardiologia Intervencionista; affirmation of value by the Canadian Association of Interventional Cardiology – Association Canadienne de Cardiologie d'Intervention). Journal of the American College of Cardiology. 2015;**65**:e7-e26

[7] 2015 SCAI/ACC/HFSA/STS clinical expert consensus statement on the use percutaneous mechanical circulatory support devices in cardiovascular care. JACC. 2015;**65**(19):2141

[8] Atkinson TM, Ohman EM, O'Neill WW, Rab T, Cigarroa JE. A practical approach to mechanical circulatory support in patients undergoing percutaneous coronary intervention: An interventional perspective. JACC: Cardiovascular Interventions. 2016;**9**(9):871-883 ISSN 1936-8798

[9] Makdisi G, Makdisi PB, Wang IW. New horizons of non-emergent use of extracorporeal membranous oxygenator support. Annals of Translational Medicine. 2016;**4**(4):76. DOI: 10.3978/j.issn.2305-5839.2016.02.04

[10] Higuchi R, Tobaru T, Hagiya K, et al. Outcomes of patients requiring extracorporeal membrane oxygenation in transcatheter aortic valve implantation: A clinical case series. Heart and Vessels. 2018;**33**:1343-1349. DOI: 10.1007/s00380-018-1183-8

[11] Trenkwalder T, Pellegrini C, Holzamer A, et al. Prophylactic ECMO during TAVI in patients with depressed left ventricular ejection fraction. Clinical Research in Cardiology.

2019;**108**:366-374. DOI: 10.1007/s00392-018-1364-6

[12] Michael S, Paul F, Jackson Simon A, Gonzalo M, Sarah A, Bannon Paul G, et al. Extracorporeal membrane oxygenation for very high-risk transcatheter aortic valve implantation. Heart, Lung & Circulation. 2014;**1-6**:1443

[13] Gopalamurugan AB, Meenakshi MS, Mohamed Abubacker R. India's first successful ECMO assisted TAVI: A strategy for 'high risk' TAVI patients. IHJ Cardiovascular Case Reports (CVCR). 2017;**1**(1):4-6, ISSN 2468-600X. DOI: 10.1016/j.ihjccr.2017.05.004

[14] Makdisi G, Makdisi PB, Wang IW. Use of extracorporeal membranous oxygenator in transcatheter aortic valve replacement. Annals of Translational Medicine. 2016;**4**:306

[15] Bedogni F et al. Trattamento transcatetere dell'insufficienza mitralica per i pazienti non eleggibili all'intervento chirurgico: Epidemiologia, diagnosi, equità di accesso ed impatto economico. Giornale Italiano di Cardiologia. 2017;**18**(2 Suppl. 1):3S-8S

[16] Mizote I, Schirmer J, Schafer U. A case of a successful Mitraclip implantation in a patient having a large coaptation gap under extracorporeal membrane oxygenation (ECMO). Catheterization and Cardiovascular Interventions. 2018;**91**:827-830

[17] Staudacher Dawid L, Christoph B, Tobias W. Severe mitral regurgitation requiring ECMO therapy treated by interventional valve reconstruction using MitraClip. Catheterization and Cardiovascular Interventions. 2015;**85**:170-175

[18] Craner RC, Carvajal T, Villablanca PA, Jahanyar J, Yang EH, Ramakrishna H. The increasing importance of percutaneous mechanical circulatory support in high-risk transcatheter coronary interventions: An evidence-based analysis. Journal of Cardiothoracic and Vascular Anesthesia. 2018;**32**:1507-1524

[19] Myat A, Patel N, Tehrani S, Banning AP, Redwood SR, Bhatt DL. Percutaneous circulatory assist devices for high-risk coronary intervention. JACC: Cardiovascular Interventions. 2015;**8**(2):229-244 ISSN 1936-8798

[20] Chieffo A, Burzotta F, Pappalardo F, Briguori C, Garbo R, Masiero G, et al. Clinical expert consensus document on the use of percutaneous left ventricular assist support devices during complex high-risk indicated PCI: Italian society of interventional cardiology working group endorsed by spanish and portuguese interventional cardiology societies. International Journal of Cardiology. 2019;**15**(293):84-90. DOI: 10.1016/j.ijcard.2019.05.065

[21] Shaukat A, Hryniewicz-Czeneszew K, Sun B, Mudy K, Wilson K, Tajti P, et al. Outcomes of extracorporeal membrane oxygenation support for complex high-risk elective percutaneous coronary interventions: A single-center experience and review of the literature. The Journal of Invasive Cardiology. 2018 Dec;**30**(12):456-460

[22] Kahaly O, Boudoulas KD. Percutaneous left ventricular assist device in high risk percutaneous coronary intervention. Journal of Thoracic Disease. 2016;**8**(3):298-302

[23] van den Brink FS, Meeljers TA, Hofma SH, van Boven AJ, Nap A, Vonk A, et al. Prophylactic veno-arterial extracorporeal membrane oxygenation in patients undergoing high-risk percutaneous coronary intervention.

Netherlands Heart Journal. 2020;**28**: 139-144

[24] Palaniswamy C, Miller MA, Reddy VY, Dukkipati SR. Hemodynamic support for ventricular tachycardia ablation. Cardiac Electrophysiology Clinics. 2017;**9**(1):141-152. DOI: 10.1016/j.ccep.2016.10.011

[25] Vallabhajosyula S, Vallabhajosyula S, Vaidya VR, Patlolla SH, Desai V, Mulpuru SK, et al. Venoarterial extracorporeal membrane oxygenation support for ventricular tachycardia ablation: A systematic review. ASAIO Journal. 2020;**66**(9):980-985. DOI: 10.1097/MAT.0000000000001125

[26] Baratto F, Pappalardo F, Oloriz T, Bisceglia C, Vergara P, Silberbauer J, et al. Extracorporeal membrane oxygenation for hemodynamic support of ventricular tachycardia ablation. Circulation. Arrhythmia and Electrophysiology. 2016;**9**(12):e004492. DOI: 10.1161/CIRCEP.116.004492

[27] Claire Watkins A, Maassel Nathan L, Mehrdad G, Dawood Murtaza Y, Pham Si M, Kon Zachary N, et al. Preoperative venoarterial extracorporeal membrane oxygenation slashes risk score in advanced structural heart disease. The Annals of Thoracic Surgery. 2018;**106**:1709-1715

[28] Brscic E, Rovero G, Sori P, Testa K, Marra S. Trattamento percutaneo di doppio vizio valvolare con sistema di ossigenazione extracorporea a membrana modificato [Percutaneous treatment of double valve defect with a modified extracorporeal membrane oxygenation system]. Giornale Italiano di Cardiologia. Rome, Italian. 2020;**21**(11):900-904. DOI: 10.1714/3455.34445. PMID: 33077997

[29] Brscic E, Rovero G, Testa K, et al. In-hospital and mid-term outcomes of ECMO support during coronary, structural or combined percutaneous cardiac interventional in a high-risk patients – A single-center experience. Cardiovascular Revascularization Medicine. 2021 Nov;**32**:63-67. DOI: 10.1016/j.carrev.2020.12.020. PMID: 33358182

Chapter 2

Venoarterial Extracorporeal Membrane Oxygenation in Cardiac Surgery

Tamer Abdalghafoor, Dina Fa Alwaheidi, Amr Salah Omar, Abdulwahid Almulla and Ali Kindawi

Abstract

Owing to the growing demands of extracorporeal membrane oxygenation (ECMO)-designated support required for severe cardiac or respiratory failure, which is both potentially reversible and unresponsive to conventional management, novel ECMO indications emerge day after day. ECMO offers unique advantageous characteristics, which are compact pump-oxygenator design, percutaneous approach, flexible cannulae, and less inflammation making the modern venoarterial ECMO an ideal miniaturized cardiopulmonary bypass. We hereby discuss the background of ECMO success to backup complex high-risk cardiac surgical procedures.

Keywords: cardiogenic shock, cardiopulmonary bypass, extracorporeal membrane oxygenation, percutaneous coronary intervention, transcutaneous aortic valve implantation

1. Introduction

Demands for venoarterial extracorporeal membrane oxygenation (VA-ECMO) are growing worldwide to support the circulation in response to cardiogenic shock (CS) [1, 2]. One of the temporary mechanical circulatory support (tMCS) devices that are employed when there is circulatory failure is VA-ECMO [3]. Since its debut in 1972, VA-ECMO has been widely used to support clinicians in a variety of complex cardiac procedures on an emergency or preventative basis, including transcutaneous aortic valve implantation (TAVI) [4], complex percutaneous coronary intervention (PCI) [5], and postcardiotomy when it is difficult to wean the cardiopulmonary bypass (CBP) machine [6]. Considering ECMO is a more compact circuit than CPB and does not require cardiotomy suction or air-blood contact, it requires less anticoagulation, which could reduce coagulopathy and minimize systemic inflammation inflammatory response [4]. Refractory CS attributable to myocarditis, acute MI, acute cor pulmonale from a major pulmonary embolism, primary transplant graft failure, postcardiotomy CS, acute exacerbation of chronic heart failure, toxic ingestions, and intractable arrhythmias are only a few examples of specific indications for VA-ECMO (**Table 1**) [5].

Common indications	Selected contraindications
Refractory cardiogenic shock secondary to:	Relative:
Acute myocardial infarction	Severe uncontrolled bleeding or when anticoagulation is contraindicated
Acute exacerbation of chronic heart failure	Severe peripheral arterial disease
Fulminant myocarditis	Aortic dissection
Massive pulmonary embolism	Prognostic score reveals poor survival benefits (modified SAVE or PREDICT VA-ECMO)
Intractable arrhythmias	Severe AI
Postcardiotomy syndrome	Absolute:
Primary transplant graft failure	Irrecoverable condition
Toxins	Unwitnessed asystole
Periprocedural Support	Goals of care not in keeping with temporary mechanical support
ECPR	

ECMO: extracorporeal membrane oxygenation; ECPR: extracorporeal cardiopulmonary resuscitation; SAVE: surviving after venoarterial ECMO trial; and VA: venoarterial.

Table 1.
Common indications and contraindications for using VA-ECMO.

This chapter will focus on the indications related to the cardiac surgery, ECPR, periprocedural support, refractory CS secondary to AMI, postcardiotomy syndrome, and other high-risk procedures that require VA-ECMO.

2. ECMO for ischemic cardiogenic shock

Despite the decline in the incidence of MI-related cardiogenic shock; myocardial infarction (MI) remains the top common cause of cardiogenic shock in more than 80% of cases [6]. Studies have shown that in the era of revascularization MI related cardiogenic shock is about 4 to 10 % [7, 8]. The largest of these studies, the SHOCK trial (Should We Emergently Revascularize Occluded Coronaries for Cardiogenic Shock) recommended an early invasive approach to treat MI-related shock state to reduce mortality. However, mortality in such devastating complications remains high approaching 30% to 50% [7–9].

The challenge in CS and refractory cardiac arrest is always how to maintain systemic circulation, and ECMO could be appropriate in this situation. In the setting of persistently poor CS outcomes and technological advances in VA-ECMO, patients treated with cardiovascular MCS have exponentially increased over the last decade [10, 11].

3. Extracorporeal cardiopulmonary resuscitation

Extracorporeal cardiopulmonary resuscitation (ECPR) refers to institution of VA-ECMO in the setting of stubborn cardiac arrest. The 2010 American Heart Association Guidelines for Cardiopulmonary Resuscitation and Emergency Cardiovascular Care stated that ECPR may be considered when spontaneous circulation interrupting time is short, appropriate resuscitation efforts, and the cardiac arrest reason is possibly reversible or could be handled with revascularization or heart transplantation [12]. The guidelines emphasize that ECPR use should be limited to special centers that got the capabilities of running this complex intervention, in the view of managerial requirements of advanced equipment and highly trained personnel.

4. ECMO for high-risk procedures

The introduction of VA-ECMO as cardiopulmonary support has paved the way for new operative indications for those patients who were previously relegated to conservative medical management. Patients with poor left ventricular function, CS with complex multivessel disease, or multiple other comorbidities now could be undergone revascularization with circulatory support of ECMO. Recent applications have shown ECMO to be potentially effective as a temporizing measure or bridge to therapeutic intervention in the setting of myocardial dysfunction and CS. Extracorporeal life support is now used in many more difficult situations due to recent advances in knowledge and familiarity. These include a number of high-risk catheter-based procedures, such as transcatheter aortic valve implantation (TAVI) and percutaneous coronary interventions (PCI) [13–15], post-infarct ventricular septal defect (PI-VSD) repair as well as surgery on the thoracoabdominal aorta, international retrievals for cardiac and respiratory failure [16], and in case of massive pulmonary thromboembolism as a bridge for embolectomy (PTE) [17].

4.1 ECMO support in high-risk percutaneous coronary intervention (HR-PCI)

Early reports of total cardiopulmonary support or cardiopulmonary bypass (CPB) during high-risk PCI were aimed at understanding the best time to initiate support, either prophylactically or to be on "standby" during the procedure. Prophylactic vs standby percutaneous CPB in HR-PCI was compared in a retrospective data analysis of 23 national registries with 569 patients. 180 patients were in the standby group and 389 patients were in the prophylactic CPB group. The procedural success rate was almost the same in both groups (88.7 % compared to 84.4 %); however, the periprocedural mortality rate was greater in the standby group (18.8 % versus 4.8 %, $p = 0.05$) [18]. Subsequent studies showed more evidence for the benefit of ECMO use in a patient with ST-segment elevation myocardial infarction (STEMI) complicated by CS unresponsive to inotropes and intra-aortic balloon pump (IABP) [19, 20].

4.1.1 Emergent PCI post myocardial infarction and cardiogenic shock

Koutouzis et al. [20] showed how ECMO assistance was used successfully and with good results during PCI in a patient with CS. Subsequently, Sheu et al. [19] recommended that patients with STEMI complicated by CS, unresponsive to inotropes and IABP placement, had lower 30-day mortality after prompt-ECMO support in the cath lab in comparison to a non-supported cohort with a similar presentation.

4.1.2 Elective PCI in high-risk patients and left main procedures

Other studies described the use of ECMO in elective, high-risk, complex PCI. In their single-center prospective investigation on the use of ECMO in these patients,

Tomasello et al. [21] published their findings. 12 consecutive patients with complicated coronary artery disease who were at high risk for surgical revascularization underwent initiation of femoro-femoral VA ECMO before the indexed PCI. All patients responded favorably to the procedure, and there was only one access site hematoma that did not need to be transfused. At the 6-month follow-up, no deaths or MI were reported. Authors proposed that ECMO might serve as a viable substitute to ensure PCI success in unsuitable surgical candidates.

4.1.3 Complicated PCI needs surgical intervention

Following percutaneous coronary intervention (PCI), complications are often successfully managed in the catheterization laboratory, but certain complications require emergent surgical intervention. One of the most dreadful, albeit rare, complications is coronary artery perforation, which occurs from 0.1% to 3.0% [22]. Patients who have developed mechanical complications produced iatrogenically during diagnostic coronary angiography (CA) and PCI are usually in critical clinical status and require immediate corrective therapy, including inotropic support and mechanical ventilation. In the worst-case scenario, mechanical assist systems such as IABP or ECMO are required in hemodynamically unstable patients [23].

4.2 High-risk TAVI and ECMO support

Although transcatheter aortic valve implantation (TAVI) is an excellent alternative procedure for high-risk patients with severe symptomatic aortic stenosis, it is often associated with life-threatening complications. TAVI can cause profound hemodynamic perturbation in the perioperative period. VA-ECMO can be used to provide cardiorespiratory support during this time, either prophylactically or emergently. Michael et al. [24] described the utilization of ECMO for patients who had significantly high mean EuroSCORE and had undergone TAVI procedures. Postoperative outcomes were broadly comparable between TAVI patients who did not require ECMO and ECMO patients who had significantly higher mean EuroSCORE. Elective use of ECMO is usually considered in patients with severe pulmonary hypertension (over 60 mmHg) and/or markedly decreased left ventricular ejection fraction (LVEF under 20%) [25]. In selected cases, it may be advocated to avoid consequences of intraoperative complications, emergency VA-ECMO associated with higher mortality [24, 26].

4.3 ECMO support for postinfarct VSD

F. Ramponi et al. reported two cases with successful use of VA-ECMO in two high-risk patients' postinfarction ventricular septal defect (VSD) and CS, with 80 % calculated mortality risk by logistic EuroSCORE. Both cases were in detrimental biventricular failure that was treated successfully with VA ECM surviving to hospital discharge [27].

4.4 ECMO and acute pulmonary embolism

The prognosis is dismal for patients who present with a massive acute pulmonary embolism (PE) exacerbated by right ventricular (RV) failure and CS [28]. Thrombolysis or embolectomy must be performed immediately, but due to logistical or hemodynamic instability, these therapeutic procedures may be postponed.

As a stabilizing measure or stepping stone to additional therapies, the use of MCS in these situations is crucial [29]. In cases of RV failure brought on by pressure overload related to pulmonary obstruction, VA-ECMO is the best course of action. Few reports showed successful use of percutaneous VA-ECMO as an adjunct to thrombolytic therapy for circulatory collapse secondary to massive PE [30]. Indeed, successful rescue therapy with ECMO has been described in several cases of life-threatening PE [31, 32], even in patients with acute cardiopulmonary collapse [33]. In some cases, complete lysis of pulmonary artery clots has been reported after a few days of ECMO and heparin treatment [31, 34, 35].

4.5 ECMO and heart transplantation

In such cases, ECMO could be used as a bridge to heart transplantation or ventricular assist device (VAD) insertion in INTERMACS class I patients or as a bridge to a decision when the prognosis is uncertain [36–40]. Patients receiving ECMO assistance must stay in the intensive care unit, and since the duration of ECMO support is shorter than that of VADs, making transplantation or switching to a VAD is more urgent [41]. The effectiveness of ECMO as a bridge therapy varies widely and is mostly influenced by the characteristics of the pre-ECMO patient and the availability of organs in situations where transplantation is the eventual goal. Additionally, primary graft failure (PGF) after heart transplantation is also treated with ECMO assistance [42, 43]. Patients with PGF who require ECMO have a poorer overall survival rate than patients without PGF. Patients with ECMO-supported PGF, however, have equivalent long-term survival to non-PGF transplant recipients who live past the immediate post-transplant period [43, 44].

5. Intraoperative VA-ECMO

Advances in ECMO technology have led to a broader application of this technique. One example is the intraoperative use of VA-ECMO instead of classical cardiopulmonary bypass (CBP).

We reported two cases where patients underwent coronary artery bypass grafting (CABG) under the support of VA-ECMO in the setting of CS complicating acute myocardial infarction [45]. One of these is a 57-year-old male with multiple comorbidities. Admitted as a case STEMI complicated by CS while undergoing primary PCI. Eventually, he needed a further support with peripheral VA-ECMO. Keeping target ACT over 180 seconds and the target a (aPTT) between 60 and 80 seconds. Coronary angiography showed left main and three-vessel CAD not amenable for PCI. The patient was kept on ECMO support and CABG was done 24hrs after. Surgery was done as beating heart while on ECMO without conversion to conventional CPB. ACT value was kept as routine above 300 seconds. Intraoperatively, VA-ECMO flow has been optimized by adjusting the inotropic support of dopamine and noradrenaline infusion to keep mean arterial pressure (MAP) above 65 mmHg. Hemostasis was achievable while keeping ACT of 180 seconds. After revascularization, intraoperative transesophageal echocardiography (TEE) showed distended left ventricle (LV) and low-velocity time integral 9 cm (VTI); therefore, we decided to keep the ECMO support after revascularization. Decannulation of VA-ECMO was done on the third postoperative day. IABP was removed on the fourth postoperative day. The patient survived to discharge.

In primary PCI, VA-ECMO is a rescue measure for CS. Cases that require emergency surgical revascularization can be carried out utilizing the ECMO circuit instead of instituting CPB circuit, and by this means, the procedure is carried out with less aortic manipulation, prompter revascularization, and less priming volumes; therefore, it needs less anticoagulation, potentially reducing coagulopathy and attenuating systemic inflammatory response [46].

6. ECMO support for postcardiotomy low cardiac output syndrome

Postcardiotomy (PC) low cardiac output syndrome is generally defined as a shock state refractory to inotropic support and\or IABP, and it can manifest as an inability to separate from CPB or persistent CS despite maximal use of pharmacological agents and\or IABP in the immediate postoperative period. It is a rare but a detrimental complication after cardiac surgery.

ECMO has been used as a salvage in such complications more than 50 years ago mainly for cardiac surgery in pediatrics but remained quiescent in adult population. However, during the last several years, ECMO is being used more and more in adult patients, particularly for postcardiotomy low cardiac output syndrome. Since its introduction to be used to support PC shock, ECMO has been a lifesaver and an important prognosis changer in such complications. It is reported that from 2007 to 2011, non-percutaneous ECMO cannulation increased 2-fold, while the use of percutaneous ECMO increased by more than 15-fold. In a study that looked at more than 9,000 ECMO patients from the Nationwide Inpatient Sample database in the US from 1998 to 2009, 4,493 cases (approximately 50%) were cannulated for cardiogenic shock in the postoperative period. In the same database, researchers observed that PC-ECMO was the most frequent ECMO indication between the years 2002 and 2011 [47]. The usage of PC-ECMO has increased over the previous ten years, according to data from the Extracorporeal Life Support Organization (ELSO) registry [48]. Despite the growing evidence and the widened use of such expensive, highly debatable yet important surgical armament. Unfortunately, data is unpowered, limited, conflicting, and highly variable.

6.1 Indications, contraindications, and cannulation of VA-ECMO

6.1.1 Indications

Currently, there is no consensus regarding when to initiate extracorporeal life support (ECLS) in the setting of postcardiotomy low cardiac output syndrome. A recent paper, the 2020 EACTS/ELSO/STS/AATS Expert Consensus on PostCardiotomy Extracorporeal Life Support in Adult Patients, represents to date the first comprehensive guideline to provide structured and clinical recommendations about the most relevant issues surrounding its application in this setting [49].

In this joint effort, the authors considered that class I indications of ECMO in the postcardiotomy setting can be summarized as follows:

- ECMO support to be initiated prior to end-organ injury or onset of anaerobic metabolism (lactate level <4mmol/l) in patients with likelihood of myocardial recovery and in the absence of uncontrollable bleeding not amenable to surgical repair [49].

- In case the likelihood of myocardial recovery is low, ECMO is recommended in patients who are eligible for long-term mechanical support or heart transplantation (LT-MCS or an HTx) [49].

In addition, timely implantation prior to severe end-organ hypoperfusion and ischemic injury represents one of the most powerful predictors of ECMO outcome, the early use of ECMO after cardiac surgery in a patient with an IABP and optimal medical therapy, with failure to wean from CPB or marginal hemodynamics also has been listed as class 1 recommendation [49]. Scoring systems were developed to prognosticate the outcomes following ECMO patients in general and mainly to help clinicians when best to avoid or consider it and it gives guidance while exploring it as an option for the families and its complications. Of these scoring tools, the survival after venoarterial-ECMO (SAVE) score has been considered one of the best predicting tools for ECMO patients in general due to its independent variable cohort; however, it was not developed to meet the special physiologic milieu of postcardiotomy patients [50].

Recently, a single-center, retrospective study that included 166 postcardiotomy CS patients supported with VA-ECMO after CABG over a 14-year period created a 6-items bedside scoring system; the REMEMBER score has been able to predict the mortality in that study cohort. It was found that older age, left main disease, inotropic score > 75, CK-MB > 130 IU/L, serum creatinine > 150 umol/L, and platelet count < 100 × 109/L were identified as pre-ECMO prognosis factors of in-hospital mortality in the REMEMBER score [51]. In this setting, again lack of evidence calls for more powerful multicenter scoring system to accurately predict the prognosis in postcardiac surgery patients requiring ECMO for PC shock.

6.1.2 Contraindications

In General, for patients in whom PC failure is felt to be reversible, all contraindications should be considered relative, except for uncontrollable bleeding not amenable for surgical correction, which is by far the only absolute contraindications for postcardiac surgery patients [49].

6.1.2.1 Relative contraindications

- Age\although patients in their 80s have been supported with success, advanced age has been linked to worse outcomes, as we mentioned earlier, careful thought of patients' appropriateness to ECMO in case they are not candidates for long-term support or heart transplantation [49].

- Comorbidities e.g., chronic lung disease, renal insufficiency, and peripheral vascular disease were also associated with poor outcomes [49].

- All degrees of aortic insufficiency need to be addressed either surgically or via transcatheter as it also affects the performance of the ECMO support by aggravating the LV distention [49].

6.1.3 Cannulation

It was found that following PC low cardiac output, approximately 40% of ECMO cannulation occurs in the operating room and 60% in the ICU [52]. As these patients' chests are already opened via sternotomy or thoracotomy; central access is an additional modality to cannulate PC patients with ECMO centrifugal pump. However, it was found that peripheral cannulation is more common than central cannulation despite its easiness in terms of the already utilized access via right atrium and aorta, the presumed as well as the gathered evidence showed higher complications in terms of mortality, bleeding, infection, and compression in case of central cannulation in comparison to the peripheral access via the femoral or the axillary sites. In a retrospective multicenter study, Mariscalco et al. compared peripheral and central VA-ECMO in 781 patients with PCS at 19 cardiac surgery centers. Concluded that central cannulation was associated with greater in-hospital mortality than peripheral cannulation, pooled unadjusted risk ratio analysis of these patients showed that patients undergoing peripheral VA-ECMO had a lower in-hospital/30-day mortality than patients undergoing central cannulation, authors stated that results did not alter after cofounders' readjustment [53].

6.1.3.1 Basic principles

6.1.3.1.1 Peripheral cannulation

It is the most frequently used access due to less complication rate and it allows sternotomy closure. It is performed via the common femoral artery and vein just below the inguinal ligament and should be above the bifurcations [54]. Arterial cannula should be adequate to supply sufficient flow to meet the patient's needs, sizes larger than 19F cannulas may be considered only when higher flow is needed and is usually rare; keeping in mind the increased vascular complications, including limb ischemia with larger cannula [55]. If feasible, some opinions prefer to place each cannula in different legs as it is thought to reduce the vascular complications associated if both cannulas are placed in the same limb. Also, some experts prefer to insert the venous cannula into the right femoral vein as it is a more direct path to the IVC and right atrium. Nowadays, the Image-guided cannulation, particularly vascular ultrasound is the standard in percutaneous approach. Fluoroscopy can be useful if available. Vascular ultrasound should be started in the short axis and longitudinal views [56].

6.1.3.1.2 Central cannulation

Although peripheral access is linked to better survival and less complication, in some instances, especially with patients with peripheral vascular disease, the adoption of central cannulation is inevitable. Utilizing the same CPB cannula in the ascending aorta and the right atrium is the most common approach. Other methods have also been described to allow sternotomy closure via tunneling the cannulas through the skin below the sternum to allow the closure, although cardiac compression and kinking of the cannula have been described as complications of this method. Cannulation configuration and strategy can be summarized as follows (**Table 2**) [49].

6.2 Management VA-ECMO

Management of patients with VA ECMO for postcardiotomy shock is more complicated than for other indications, as surgical patients are usually sicker with many other comorbidities and an already injured heart. Arterial blood gases, lactates, mixed venous oxygen saturation (SvO2), and urine output are all indicators to follow and

	Advantages	Disadvantages
Central (aortic\ atrial)	• More efficient drainage via antegrade flow • Direct access via established surgical site with possibility of sternotomy closure. • Avoids harlequin syndrome	• Opened chest* • More bleeding • Re-sternotomy is mandatory to decannulate
Peripheral		
Percutaneous femoral artery	• Can be done Bedside • Avoids surgical incisions so less bleeding • Less sepsis • Can be switched to VAD implant easily	• High limb ischemia complications • LV afterload due to retrograde flow • LV venting cannot be easily achieved • Not suitable for long-lasting support
Open femoral artery	• Appropriate cannulation sites via Direct visualization of femoral vessels • Less bleeding • Avoids sternotomy	• limb ischemia complications • LV afterload due to retrograde flow • LV venting cannot be easily achieved • Not suitable for long-lasting support
Pseudo-central		
Axillary\ Subclavian	• Long lasting support • Easy patient mobilization • Avoidance of Harlequin (North/South) Syndrome	• Time-consuming • Upper limb vascular complications Lower ECMO flow

**Closed chest is accessible; however, cardiac compression is likely with central approach.*

Table 2.
Cannulation configuration and strategy summary.

manage the ECMO patients. Close clinical follow-up using echocardiogram is also crucial to determine the overall cardiac function, right ventricular (RV) function in case RV is not supported, velocity time interval (VTI) are important parameters as well [49].

6.2.1 Sternotomy wound management

Despite the cannulation site, sternotomy wounds should always be closed to minimize bleeding and also to reduce infections. In case of peripheral cannulation, this can be easily achieved as cannulae are already apart from the wound, but central cannulation might add complexity to the closure. Some have proposed tunneling techniques to divert the cannula away from the wound although it has been shown that it might cause cardiac compression by the cannula themselves in case of subxiphoid tunneling, other tunneling techniques with less compression included externalization through the intercostal spaces, tunneling into the neck to the jugular area, or the anastomosis to prosthetic grafts, which is usually utilized in aortic surgery [57, 58].

6.2.2 Leg perfusion

In case of femoral cannulation, many ways have been adopted to reduce ischemic and vascular complications such as adopting the open technique as possible, using a smaller cannula, and using vascular graft instead of direct femoral cannulation, but most importantly using distal perfusion cannula to perfuse the cannulated leg. This cannula is then connected with a side way to the arterial cannula and its flow can be monitored using a sensor to ensure optimal leg perfusion. Moreover, continuous daily pulse monitoring should be ensured [49].

6.2.3 Flow management

Determining how much flow is best to achieve optimal peripheral perfusion with some heart ejection remains unclear. Some have argued that allowing the supported heart to eject is better than full support in terms that it prevents the blood stasis as well as the dilatation [59–61]; however, as mentioned earlier, PC patients are different as the heart is already damaged so allowing the heart to eject might add extra workload [62].

6.2.4 Left ventricular distention

Although infrequent, LV distention is one of the major issues facing the supported heart while on ECMO regardless of the site of the cannulation as retrograde ECMO flow adds more on the afterload, which can be hazardous for an already dysfunctional ventricle, which is usually the case in PC patients. Another important mechanism, it has been postulated that while on ECMO the aortic valve might exhibit a protracted closure due to the impedance of the forward flow, which causes blood stasis, blood pooling, LV wall tension, and LV workload even in the absence of poor myocardium. For that, several clinical studies have shown that IABP might be beneficial in eliminating the LV distention by restoring AV opening and reducing forward flow impendence [63]. However, in extreme cases of LV dysfunction, IABP might not be enough to alleviate the distention, in such cases more invasive methods should intervene such as direct cannulation of the LV through the apex, surgical or percutaneous cannulation of the pulmonary artery may be considered for indirect LV unloading as well. Trans-aortic devices such as impella and impella RP have also shown great benefit in this setting. Another approach including trans-septal approach surgically or percutaneously has been also used [64]. The true prevalence of LV distention and its clinical impact remains unproven, also the need for LV venting and whether its prophylactic implementation is useful is unknown.

6.2.5 Anticoagulation

The most adopted practice for PC ECMO is to partially reverse with half dose protamine and then wait for 24-48hrs for full heparin administration after excluding major bleeding. As mediastinal collection can be one of the most associated complications after ECMO institution as ECMO itself can exacerbate coagulopathy, management should be directed toward a balance between bleeding management with product transfusion and medication in facing clot formation prevention in the circuit [65–67]. Unfractionated heparin remains an antithrombotic agent of choice for anticoagulation in case of PC ECMO as per the ELSO guidelines. Although monitoring has not been standardized yet, it is recommended that either ACT targeting a level of 180–200s or aPTT up to 50–80s is accepted [68, 69]. In any case of prolonged use of heparin, the possibility of HITT occurrence is likely, in such case direct thrombin inhibitors (DTI) can be used, such as bivalirudin should be used, as an alternative. However, extra caution should be kept given the very short half-life of bivalirudin so the likelihood of developing clots can be life-threatening [70].

6.2.6 Intensive care monitoring

Systematic clinical examination along with physiological and laboratory monitoring with close adjustment of ECMO setting should be implemented. Monitoring of all peripheral arterial saturation should be done for early detection of harlequin syndrome in case of uneven distribution of saturation. Recognizing early signs of infection and early start of empiric antibiotics is crucial to avoid the burden of septic shock occurrence [49].

Timely detection of brain injury is considered an important aspect to consider while in ICU monitoring, and it has been shown that EEG and near-infrared spectroscopy (NIRS) play an important diagnostic and prognostic role in the timely detection of acute brain injury [71, 72]. Confirming the diagnosis with CT is also encouraged despite the complexity of transportation while on ECMO. Nonetheless, transesophageal echocardiographic (TEE) is an important tool to assess the overall cardiac function, cannula positions, and right ventricular dynamics and to guide the suitability of weaning. In our institute, we do not use the swan-Ganz catheter, but it might be useful in few cases to guide management.

6.3 Weaning from VA-ECMO

The consideration for weaning EMCO exists when absence of specific decompensation factors like supraventricular arrhythmia or severe septic shock could be managed. Recovery of pulsatile arterial waveform for at least 24 h, the patient should be hemodynamically stable, with mean arterial pressure more than 60 mmHg in the absence or reducing doses of inotropes and/or vasopressors [73]. Finally, pulmonary function should be adequate with PaO2/FiO2 more than 200 mmHg [74]. It is unlikely to start weaning trial in the first 72 hours of initiation [75]. Weaning trial starts usually with reducing ECMO blood flow, which eventually causes right ventricular preload increase and LV afterload reduction, therefore myocardial function could be assessed [76]. Patients should have a pulsatile flow with a minimum ECMO flow of 1–1.5 L/min [77]. If mean blood pressure is reduced below 60 mmHg the trial should be abandoned. The echocardiographic criteria favoring successful weaning include LVEF of more than 20–25 %. Patients successfully weaned had aortic velocity time integral above 10 cm, and TDSa of at least 6 cm/s at minimal ECMO flow support [75].

6.4 Complications and early and long-term outcomes

Despite the exponential increase in ECMO use, PC ECMO is still in the beginning although enormous improvement in ECMO cannulation and management; successful weaning from PC ECMO varies greatly among the published series from 30% to 70%, and the survival to discharge is even much lower [78]. In the most recent ELSO registry, survival for discharge for overall ECMO cases for cardiogenic shock is 50 % [79]. So far, no RCTs have been deployed to illustrate the real survival benefit or even the quality of life in the long term. Based on the most recent report from the ELSO registry, there has been a gradual decline in the survival after PC-ECMO, as low as 15% survival in some analyses [80]. Overall, bleeding is the most frequent complication occurring in up to 90% of patients as described in some series. Other anticoagulation-related complications also can happen such as heparin-induced thrombocytopenia, intracranial bleeding, and hemolysis. Other complications include high inflammatory markers manifested as inflammatory response that is like that in systemic inflammatory response syndrome, causing an increased risk of thrombosis, infections, sepsis, and end-organ damage thus worsening patient outcomes, steroids have been used as a prophylactic agent and shown to reduce it; However, it did not affect the overall mortality [81, 82]. The prevalence of infection during ECMO is 10% to 12%, with Staphylococcus aureus, Candida, Enterobacteriaceae, and Pseudomonas aeruginosa being the most common bloodstream infective organisms. ECMO site infections are common as well, so special care for ECMO wounds and early recognition are needed. Regular cultures could be done if an infection is suspected, especially with prolonged ECMO use [83]. Limb ischemia is a major vascular complication associated with ECMO, especially the peripherally cannulated; limbs should be frequently monitored by duplex ultrasound also ECMO flow through the distal perfusion cannula should be maintained [84].

6.4.1 Predicting mortality and quality of life

Predictors for PC ECMO outcome have been studied in many papers, as mentioned earlier scoring systems were also deficient and limited not to authentically predicting outcomes after cardiac surgery. One of the pre-ECMO factors, ECPR was found to have a strong negative predictor of survival in several series [85, 86]. Others have demonstrated that blood lactate level prior to ECMO and up to 48 hours after ECMO initiation is strong predictor value for survival [87]. Early initiation of ECMO has been shown to result in higher survival rates and decrease the dosage of vasoactive drugs by increasing cardiac output and rapidly decreasing arterial lactate levels after cardiovascular surgery [88].

The CESAR trial showed a significant increase in survival without severe disability when ECMO was used instead of conventional ventilation [89].

It is been demonstrated in many series that renal and liver failure, respiratory failure, and the duration of ECMO support are also strong negative predictor factors to affect ECMO outcome [90, 91]. Despite the advances in its use, the ethical and economic implications of ECMO are enormous for both patients and the health system. Psychological distress and memory problems were described in some analyses for post-ECMO survivors. Unfortunately, the long outcome of VA-ECMO survivors remains under investigation. Most studies concentrate on treatment outcomes and survival-to-hospital discharge. The outcomes of 138 patients treated with ECMO for cardiogenic shock are related to acute myocardial infarction. Burrell et al. determined that good long-term survival could be achieved following ECMO, observing 79% survival at 12 months. Survival data are available for only 66% of patients at 24 months [92]. Ørbo et al. identified 30 (41%) of 74 ECMO survivors in Norway and surveyed 23 survivors, with 40% of respondents reporting some degree of restriction in everyday activities and depression in 35% of cases [93]. According to ELSO's data registry, CS was the most common cardiac indication in adult patients with over 2000 runs and with successful ECMO explanations in 56% of cases and an overall 42% survival-to-discharge in 2016 in participating centers. Although not evidenced by powered data, overall long-term outcomes for survivors can be promising especially with improved indications and guidelines.

7. Conclusions

Complex cardiac surgical procedures in high-risk patients may require extending the medical support to a mechanical one. VA-ECMO could offer additional advantages over CBP to support the circulation during CABG surgery in patients with complex coronary anatomy and unstable hemodynamics, with added hemodynamic and economic value.

Conflict of interest

The author(s) declared no potential conflicts of interest with respect to the research, authorship, and/or publication of this work.

Author details

Tamer Abdalghafoor[1]*, Dina Fa Alwaheidi[1], Amr Salah Omar[1], Abdulwahid Almulla[2] and Ali Kindawi[1]

1 Department of Cardiothoracic Surgery, Heart Hospital, Hamad Medical Corporation, Doha, Qatar

2 Department of Cardiothoracic Anaesthesia and Intensive Care, Heart Hospital, Doha, Qatar

*Address all correspondence to: tamerabedalghafoor@hotmail.com

References

[1] Stretch R, Sauer CM, Yuh DD, et al. National trends in the utilization of short-term mechanical circulatory support: Incidence, outcomes, and cost analysis. Journal of the American College of Cardiology. 2014;**64**:1407-1415

[2] Cavarocchi NC. Introduction to extracorporeal membrane oxygenation. Critical Care Clinics. 2017;**33**:763-766

[3] Keebler ME, Haddad EV, Choi CW, et al. Venoarterial extracorporeal membrane oxygenation in cardiogenic shock. JACC Heart Failure. 2018;**6**:503-516

[4] Makdisi G, Makdisi PB, Wang IW. Use of extracorporeal membranous oxygenator in transcatheter aortic valve replacement. Annals of Translational Medicine. 2016;**4**:306

[5] Eckman PM et al. Veno-arterial extracorporeal membrane oxygenation for cardiogenic shock: An introduction for the busy clinician. Circulation. 2019;**140**(24):2019-2037

[6] van Diepen S, Katz JN, Albert NM, Henry TD, Jacobs AK, Kapur NK, et al. American Heart Association Council on Clinical Cardiology; Council on Cardiovascular and Stroke Nursing; Council on Quality of Care and Outcomes Research; and Mission: Lifeline. Contemporary management of cardiogenic shock: A scientific statement from the American Heart Association. Circulation. 2017;**136**:e232-e268. DOI: 10.1161/CIR.0000000000000525

[7] Aissaoui N, Puymirat E, Juilliere Y, Jourdain P, Blanchard D, Schiele F, et al. Fifteen-year trends in the management of cardiogenic shock and associated 1-year mortality in elderly patients with acute myocardial infarction: The FAST-MI programme. European Journal of Heart Failure. 2016;**18**:1144-1152

[8] Kolte D, Khera S, Aronow WS, Mujib M, Palaniswamy C, Sule S, et al. Trends in incidence, management, and outcomes of cardiogenic shock complicating ST-elevation myocardial infarction in the United States. Journal of American Heart Association. 2014;**3**:e000590

[9] Thiele H, Zeymer U, Neumann FJ, Ferenc M, Olbrich HG, Hausleiter J, et al. Intraaortic Balloon Pump in cardiogenic shock II (IABP-SHOCK II) trial investigators. Intra-aortic balloon counterpulsation in acute myocardial infarction complicated by cardiogenic shock (IABP-SHOCK II): Final 12 month results of a randomised, open-label trial. Lancet. 2013;**382**:1638-1645. DOI: 10.1016/S0140-6736(13)61783-3

[10] Stretch R, Sauer CM, Yuh DD, Bonde P. National trends in the utilization of short-term mechanical circulatory support: Incidence, outcomes, and cost analysis. Journal of the American College of Cardiology. 2014;**64**:1407-1415. DOI: 10.1016/j.jacc.2014.07.958

[11] Thiagarajan RR, Barbaro RP, Rycus PT, Mcmullan DM, Conrad SA, Fortenberry JD, et al. ELSO member centers. Extracorporeal Life Support Organization Registry International Report 2016. ASAIO Journal. 2017;**63**:60-67

[12] Cave DM, Gazmuri RJ, Otto CW, Nadkarni VM, Cheng A, et al. Part 7: CPR techniques and devices: 2010 American Heart Association Guidelines for Cardiopulmonary Resuscitation

and Emergency Cardiovascular Care. Circulation. 2010;**122**:S720-S728

[13] Spina R, Forrest AP, Adams MR, Wilson MK, Ng MK, Vallely MP. Veno-arterial extracorporeal membrane oxygenation for high-risk cardiac catheterisation procedures. Heart, Lung & Circulation. 2010;**19**(12):736-741

[14] Vallely MP, Wilson MK, Adams M, Ng MKC. How to set up a successful TAVI program. Annals of Cardiothoracic Surgery. 2012;**1**(2):185-189

[15] Ramponi F, Yan TD, Vallely MP, Wilson MK. Total percutaneous cardiopulmonary bypass with Perclose ProGlide. Interactive Cardiovascular and Thoracic Surgery. 2011;**13**(1):86-88

[16] Forrest P, Cheong JY, Vallely MP, Torzillo PJ, Hendel PN, Wilson MK, et al. International retrieval of adults on extracorporeal membrane oxygenation support. Anaesthesia and Intensive Care. 2011;**39**(6):1082-1085

[17] Ramponi F, Wilson MK, Vedelago J, Bayfield MS. Catastrophic pulmonary and paradoxical embolism. ANZ Journal of Surgery. 2011;**81**(11):843-844

[18] Teirstein PS, Vogel RA, Dorros G, et al. Prophylactic versus standby cardiopulmonary support for high risk percutaneous transluminal coronary angioplasty. Journal of the American College of Cardiology. 1993;**21**:590-596

[19] Sheu JJ, Tsai TH, Lee FY, et al. Early extracorporeal membrane oxygenator-assisted primary percutaneous coronary intervention improved 30-day clinical outcomes in patients with ST-segment elevation myocardial infarction complicated with profound cardiogenic shock. Critical Care Medicine. 2010;**38**: 1810-1817

[20] Koutouzis M, Kolsrud O, Albertsson P. et al, Percutaneous coronary intervention facilitated by extracorporeal membrane oxygenation support in a patient with cardiogenic shock. Hellenic Journal of Cardiology. 2010;**51**:271-274

[21] Tomasello SD, Boukhris M, Ganyukov V. et al, Outcome of extracorporeal membrane oxygenation support for complex high-risk elective percutaneous coronary interventions: A single-center experience. Heart. 2015;**44**:309-313

[22] Ellis SG, Ajluni S, Arnold AZ, Popma JJ, Bittl JA, Eigler NL, et al. Increased coronary perforation in the new device era: Incidence, classification, management, and outcome. Circulation. 1994;**90**:2725-2730

[23] Verevkin A, von Aspern K, Leontyev S, Lehmann S, Borger MA, Davierwala PM. Early and long-term outcomes in patients undergoing cardiac surgery following iatrogenic injuries during percutaneous coronary intervention. Journal of the American Heart Association. 2019;**8**(1):e010940

[24] Seco M, Forrest P, Jackson SA, Martinez G, Andvik S, Bannon PG, et al. Extracorporeal membrane oxygenation for very high-risk transcatheter aortic valve implantation. Heart, Lung & Circulation. 2014;**23**(10):957-962

[25] Uehara K, Minakata K, Saito N, Imai M, Daijo H, Nakatsu T, et al. Use of extracorporeal membrane oxygenation in complicated transcatheter aortic valve replacement. General Thoracic and Cardiovascular Surgery. 2017;**65**(6):329-336

[26] Husser O, Holzamer A, Philipp A, Nunez J, Bodi V, Müller T, et al. Emergency and prophylactic use of miniaturized veno-arterial

extracorporeal membrane oxygenation in transcatheter aortic valve implantation. Catheterization and Cardiovascular Interventions. 2013;**82**(4):E542-E551

[27] Sangalli F, Patroniti N, Pesenti A, editors. ECMO-Extracorporeal Life Support in Adults. Milan: Springer; 2014

[28] Torbicki A, Perrier A, Konstantinides S, Agnelli G, Galiè N, Pruszczyk P, et al. Guidelines on the diagnosis and management of acute pulmonary embolism: The Task Force for the Diagnosis and Management of Acute Pulmonary Embolism of the European Society of Cardiology (ESC). European Heart Journal. 2008;**29**(18):2276-2315

[29] Norita H, Ohteki H, Hisanou R. Emergency pulmonary embolectomy for massive pulmonary embolism. Journal of Japan College of Angiology. 1994;**34**:3-9

[30] Misawa Y, Fuse K, Yamaguchi T, Saito T, Konishi H. Mechanical circulatory assist for pulmonary embolism. Perfusion. 2000;**15**(6):527-529H

[31] Omar HR, Miller J, Mangar D, Camporesi EM. Experience with extracorporeal membrane oxygenation in massive and submassive pulmonary embolism in a tertiary care center. The American Journal of Emergency Medicine. 2013;**31**:1616-1617

[32] Deehring R, Kiss AB, Garrett A, Hillier AG. Extracorporeal membrane oxygenation as a bridge to surgical embolectomy in acute fulminant pulmonary embolism. The American Journal of Emergency Medicine. 2006;**24**:879-880

[33] Hsieh PC, Wang SS, Ko WJ, Han YY, Chu SH. Successful resuscitation of acute massive pulmonary embolism with extracorporeal membrane oxygenation and open embolectomy. The Annals of Thoracic Surgery. 2001;**72**:266-267

[34] Maggio P, Hemmila M, Haft J, Bartlett R. Extracorporeal life support for massive pulmonary embolism. The Journal of Trauma. 2007;**62**:570-576

[35] Davies MJ, Arsiwala SS, Moore HM, Kerr S, Sosnowski AW, et al. Extracorporeal membrane oxygenation for the treatment of massive pulmonary embolism. The Annals of Thoracic Surgery. 1995;**60**:1801-1803

[36] Arpesella G, Loforte A, Mikus E, Mikus PM. Extracorporeal membrane oxygenation for primary allograft failure. Transplantation Proceedings. 2008;**40**:3596-3597

[37] Chen YS, Ko WJ, Chi NH, Wu IH, Huang SC, et al. Risk factor screening scale to optimize treatment for potential heart transplant candidates under extracorporeal membrane oxygenation. American Journal of Transplantation. 2004;**4**:1818-1825

[38] Chou NK, Luo JM, Chi NH, Wu IH, Huang SC, et al. Extracorporeal membrane oxygenation and Thoratec pneumatic ventricular assist devices as double bridge to heart transplantation. Transplantation Proceedings. 2012;**44**:878-880

[39] Chung JC, Tsai PR, Chou NK, Chi NH, Wang SS, et al. Extracorporeal membrane oxygenation bridge to adult heart transplantation. Clinical Transplantation. 2010;**24**:375-380

[40] McMurray JJ, Adamopoulos S, Anker SD, Auricchio A, Bohm M, et al. ESC guidelines for the diagnosis and treatment of acute and chronic heart failure 2012: The Task Force for the Diagnosis and Treatment of Acute and Chronic Heart Failure 2012 of

the European Society of Cardiology. Developed in collaboration with the Heart Failure Association (HFA) of the ESC. European Heart Journal. 2012;**33**:1787-1847

[41] Combes A, Leprince P, Luyt CE, Bonnet N, Trouillet JL, et al. Outcomes and long-term quality-of-life of patients supported by extracorporeal membrane oxygenation for refractory cardiogenic shock. Critical Care Medicine. 2008;**36**:1404-1411

[42] D'Alessandro C, Aubert S, Golmard JL, Praschker BL, Luyt CE, et al. Extra-corporeal membrane oxygenation temporary support for early graft failure after cardiac transplantation. European Journal of Cardio-Thoracic Surgery. 2010;**37**:343-349

[43] D'Alessandro C, Golmard JL, Barreda E, Laali M, Makris R, et al. Predictive risk factors for primary graft failure requiring temporary extra-corporeal membrane oxygenation support after cardiac transplantation in adults. European Journal of Cardio-Thoracic Surgery. 2011;**40**:962-969

[44] Marasco SF, Vale M, Pellegrino V, Preovolos A, Leet A, et al. Extracorporeal membrane oxygenation in primary graft failure after heart transplantation. The Annals of Thoracic Surgery. 2010;**90**:1541-1546

[45] Abdalghafoor T, Shoman B, Salah Omar A, Shouman Y, Almulla A. Urgent coronary artery bypass graft surgery supported by veno-arterial extracorporeal membrane oxygenation: A report of two cases. Perfusion. 2021;**31**:0267

[46] Makdisi G, Makdisi PB, Wang IW. Use of extracorporeal membranous oxygenator in transcatheter aortic valve replacement. Annals of Translational Medicine. 2016;**4**:306

[47] Maxwell BG, Powers AJ, Sheikh AY, et al. Resource use trends in extracorporeal membrane oxygenation in adults: An analysis of the Nationwide Inpatient Sample 1998-2009. Journal of Thoracic Cardiovascular Surgery. 2014;**148**:416

[48] Whitman GJR. Extracorporeal membrane oxygenation for the treatment of postcardiotomy shock. The Journal of Thoracic and Cardiovascular Surgery. 2017;**153**:95-101

[49] Lorusso R, Whitman G, Milojevic M, Raffa G, McMullan DM, Boeken U, et al. 2020 EACTS/ELSO/STS/AATS expert consensus on post-cardiotomy extracorporeal life support in adult patients. European Journal of Cardio-Thoracic Surgery. 2021;**59**(1):12-53

[50] Schmidt M, Burrell A, Roberts L, Bailey M, Sheldrake J, Rycus PT, et al. Predicting survival after ECMO for refractory cardiogenic shock: The survival after veno-arterial-ECMO (SAVE)-score. European Heart Journal. 2015;**36**(33):2246-2256

[51] Wang L, Yang F, Wang X, Xie H, Fan E, Ogino M, et al. Predicting mortality in patients undergoing VA-ECMO after coronary artery bypass grafting: The REMEMBER score. Critical Care. 2019;**23**(1):11

[52] Rastan AJ, Dege A, Mohr M, Doll N, Falk V, Walther T, et al. Early and late outcomes of 517 consecutive adult patients treated with extracorporeal membrane oxygenation for refractory postcardiotomy cardiogenic shock. Journal of Thoracic Cardiovascular Surgery. 2010;**139**(2):302

[53] Mariscalco G, Salsano A, Fiore A, Dalén M, Ruggieri VG, Saeed D, et al. Peripheral versus central extracorporeal membrane oxygenation for post

cardiotomy shock: Multicenter registry, systematic review, and meta-analysis. The Journal of Thoracic and Cardiovascular Surgery. 2020;**160**:1207-1216. DOI: 10.1016/j.jtcvs.2019.10.078

[54] Raffa GM, Kowalewski M, Brodie D, et al. Meta-analysis of peripheral or central extracorporeal membrane oxygenation in post cardiotomy and non-post cardiotomy shock. The Annals of Thoracic Surgery. 2019;**107**:311-321

[55] Brogan T et al. ELSO Specialist Manual. 4th ed. Ann Arbor, MI: Extracorporeal Life Support Organization (ELSO); 2018

[56] Weymann A, Sabashnikov A, Patil NP, Mohite PN, Zych B, Garcia Saez D, et al. Minimally invasive access for central extracorporeal life support: How we do it. Artificial Organs. 2015 Feb;**39**(2):179-181

[57] Lorusso R, Bidar E, Natour E, Heuts S. Minimally invasive management of central extracorporeal membrane oxygen- ation. Journal of Cardiac Surgery. 2019;**34**:131-133

[58] Rupprecht H, Lunz D, Philipp A, Lubnow M, Schmid C. Pitfalls in percutaneous ECMO cannulation. Heart Lung Vessel. 2015;**7**:320-326

[59] Greco G, Cortinovis B, Avalli L. Left ventricular rest and unloading during VA ECMO. In: Sangalli F, Patroniti N, Pesenti A, et al., editors. ECMO-Extracorporeal Life Support in Adults. Milan: Springer Milan; 2014. pp. 193-206

[60] Ostadal P, Mlcek M, Kruger A, et al. Increasing venoarterial extracorporeal membrane oxygenation flow negatively affects left ventricular performance in a porcine model of cardiogenic shock. Journal of Translational Medicine. 2015;**13**:266

[61] Aissaoui N, Luyt CE, Leprince P, et al. Predictors of successful extracorporeal membrane oxygenation (ECMO) weaning after assistance for refractory cardiogenic shock. Intensive Care Medicine. 2011;**37**:1738-1745

[62] Pappalardo F, Montisci A. Veno-arterial extracorporeal membrane oxygenation (VA-ECMO) in postcardiotomy cardiogenic shock: How much pump flow is enough? Journal of Thoracic Disease. 2016;**8**:E1444-E1448

[63] Weber KT, Janicki JS. A review of physiology principles, clinical results and device safety. The Annals of Thoracic Surgery. 1974;**17**:602-636

[64] Meani P, Gelsomino S, Natour E, Johnson DM, Rocca HB, Pappalardo F, et al. Modalities and effects of left ventricle unloading on extracorporeal life support: A review of the current literature. European Journal of Heart Failure. 2017;**19**:84-91

[65] Tauber H, Ott H, Streif W, Weigel G, Loacker L, Fritz J, et al. Extracorporeal membrane oxygenation induces short-term loss of high-molecular-weight von Willebrand factor mul- timers. Anesthesia and Analgesia. 2015;**120**:730-736

[66] Nair P, Hoechter DJ, Buscher H, Venkatesh K, Whittam S, Joseph J, et al. Prospective observational study of hemostatic alterations during adult extracorporeal membrane oxygen- ation (ECMO) using point-of-care thromboelastometry and platelet aggregometry. Journal of Cardiothoracic and Vascular Anesthesia. 2015;**29**:288-296

[67] Repesse X, Au SM, Brechot N, Trouillet JL, Leprince P, Chastre J, et al. Recombinant factor VIIa for uncontrollable bleeding in

patients with extracorporeal membrane oxygenation: Report on 15 cases and literature review. Critical Care. 2013;**17**:R55

[68] Bembea MM, Annich G, Rycus P, Oldenburg G, Berkowitz I, Pronovost P. Variability in anticoagulation management of patients on extracorporeal membrane oxygenation: An international survey. Pediatric Critical Care Medicine. 2013;**14**:e77-e84

[69] Atallah S, Liebl M, Fitousis K, Bostan F, Masud F. Evalua- tion of the activated clotting time and activated partial thromboplastin time for the monitoring of heparin in adult extracorporeal membrane oxygenation patients. Perfusion. 2014;**29**:456-461

[70] Ranucci M. Bivalirudin and post-cardiotomy ECMO: A word of caution. Critical Care. 2012;**16**:427

[71] Sinnah F, Dalloz M-A, Magalhaes E, Wanono R, Neuville M, Smonig R, et al. Early electroencephalography findings in cardiogenic shock patients treated by venoarterial extra- corporeal membrane oxygenation. Critical Care Medicine. 2018;**46**:e389-e394

[72] Cho SM, Ziai W, Mayasi Y, Gusdon AM, Creed J, Sharrock M, et al. Noninvasive neurological monitoring in extracorporeal membrane oxygenation. ASAIO Journal. 2020;**66**:388-393

[73] Ghodsizad A, Koerner MM, Brehm CE, El-Banayosy A. The role of extracorporeal membrane oxygenation circulatory support in the crash and burn patient: From implantation to weaning. Current Opinion in Cardioloy. 2014;**29**:275-280

[74] Schmidt M, Zogheib E, Roze H, Repesse X, Lebreton G, Luyt CE, et al. The preserve mortality risk score and analysis of long-term outcomes after extracorporeal membrane oxygenation for severe acute respiratory distress syndrome. Intensive Care Medicine. 2013;**39**:1704-1713

[75] Aissaoui N, El-Banayosy A, Combes A. How to wean a patient from veno-arterial extracorporeal membrane oxygenation. Intensive Care Medicine. 2015;**41**(5):902-905

[76] Aissaoui N, Guerot E, Combes A, Delouche A, Chastre J, Leprince P, et al. Two-dimensional strain rate and Doppler tissue myocardial velocities: Analysis by echocardiography of hemodynamic and functional changes of the failed left ventricle during different degrees of extracorporeal life support. Journal of the American Society of Echocardiography. 2012;**25**:632-640

[77] 2c)Trouillet JL, Leger P, Pavie A, Diebold B, Chastre J, Combes A. Predictors of successful extracorporeal membrane oxygenation (ECMO) weaning after assistance for refractory cardiogenic shock. Intensive Care Medicine. 2011;**37**:1738-1174

[78] Bakhtiary F, Keller H, Dogan S, et al. Venoarterial extracorporeal membrane oxygenation for treatment of cardiogenic shock: Clinical experiences in 45 adult patients. The Journal of Thoracic and Cardiovascular Surgery. 2008;**135**:382-388

[79] Magovern GJ Jr, Magovern JA, Benckart DH, et al. Extracorporeal membrane oxygenation: Preliminary results in patients with postcar- diotomy cardiogenic shock. Annals of Thoracic Surgery. 1994;**57**:1462-1468

[80] Saxena P, Neal J, Joyce LD, et al. Extracorporeal membrane oxygen- ation support in postcardiotomy elderly

patients: The Mayo Clinic experience. The Annals of Thoracic Surgery. 2015;**99**:2053-2060

[81] Dieleman JM, van Paassen J, van Dijk D, et al. Prophylactic corti-costeroids for cardiopulmonary bypass in adults. Cochrane Database of Systematic Reviews. 2011;**5**:CD005566

[82] Dieleman JM, Nierich AP, Rosseel PM, et al. Intraoperative high-dose dexamethasone for cardiac surgery: A randomized controlled trial. Journal of the American Medical Association. 2012;**308**(17):1761-1767

[83] Biffi S, di Bella S, Scaravilli V, et al. Infections during extracorporeal membrane oxygenation: Epidemiology, risk factors, pathogenesis and prevention. International Antimicrobial Agents. 2017;**50**(1):9-16

[84] Bonicolini E, Martucci G, Simons J, et al. Limb ischemia in peripheral veno-arterial extracorporeal membrane oxygenation: A narrative re- view of incidence, prevention, monitoring, and treatment. Critical Care. 2019;**23**:266

[85] Distelmaier K, Schrutka L, Binder C, et al. Cardiac arrest does not affect survival in post-operative cardiovascular surgery patients undergoing extracorporeal membrane oxygenation. Resuscitation. 2016;**104**:24-27

[86] Mazzeffi MA, Sanchez PG, Herr D, et al. Outcomes of extracorporeal cardiopulmonary resuscitation for refractory cardiac arrest in adult cardiac surgery patients. The Journal of Thoracic and Cardiovascular Surgery. 2016;**152**:1133-1139

[87] Fux T, Holm M, Corbascio M, Lund LH, van der Linden J. Venoarterial extracorporeal membrane oxygenation for postcardiotomy shock: Risk factors for mortality. The Journal of Thoracic and Cardiovascular Surgery. 2018;**156**:1894-1902

[88] Ziganshin BA, Elefteriades JA. Deep hypothermic circulatory arrest. Annals of Cardiothoracic Surgery. 2013;**2**:303

[89] Peek GJ, Mugford M, Tiruvoipati R, et al. Efficacy and economic assessment of conventional ventilatory support versus extra-corporeal membrane oxygenation for severe adult respiratory failure (CESAR). Lancet. 2009;**372**:1351

[90] Slottosch I, Liakopoulos O, Kuhn E, et al. Outcomes after peripheral extracorporeal membrane oxygenation therapy for postcardiotomy cardiogenic shock: A single-center experience. The Journal of Surgical Research. 2013;**181**:e47-e55

[91] Unosawa S, Sezai A, Hata M, et al. Long-term outcomes of patients undergoing extracoporeal membrane oxygenation for refractory post-cardiotomy cardiogenic shock. Surgery Today. 2013;**43**:264-270

[92] Burrell AJC, Pellegrino VA, Wolfe R, Wong WK, Cooper DJ, Kaye DM, et al. Long-term survival of adults with cardi-ogenic shock after venoarterial extracorporeal membrane oxygenation. Journal of Critical Care. 2015;**30**:949-956

[93] Ørbo MC, Karlsen SF, Pedersen EP, Hermansen SE, Rønning PB, Nergaard KA, et al. Health-related quality of life after extracorporeal membrane oxygenation: A single centre's experience. ESC Heart Failure. 2019;**6**:701-710

Chapter 3

Extracorporeal Membrane Oxygenation for the Support of Adults with Acute Myocarditis

Aggeliki Gkouziouta

Abstract

Myocarditis is an inflammatory disease of the myocardium diagnosed through a combination of histological, immunological and immunohistochemical criteria. Its clinical presentation varies from an acute coronary-like symptoms to heart failure. Diagnostic workup includes elevated biomarkers, ECG and echocardiographic findings. Cardiac magnetic resonance is the most important examination providing information on both ventricular function and tissue characterization. However, in the case of critically ill patients, CMR should be replaced with endomyocardial biopsy (EMB) which remains the gold standard in myocarditis diagnosis. EMB provides information on both the etiology and prognosis thus affecting the therapeutic approach to the patient. For example, virus positive myocarditis benefits from antiviral treatment while in virus negative ones, immunosuppression is more appropriate. Mechanical circulatory support (MCS) is often necessary in patients presenting with cardiogenic shock. MCS includes intra-aortic balloon pump, temporary percutaneous or even surgically implanted ventricular assist devices and extracorporeal membrane oxygenation (ECMO). ECMO essentially bypasses the heart and provides adequate oxygenation to peripheral organs. Due to the increased afterload under ECMO support, it seems reasonable to be combined with intra-aortic balloon pump or percutaneous VAD implantation to promote left ventricular unloading and potential recovery.

Keywords: myocarditis, cardiogenic shock, ecmosupport, extracorporeal membrane oxygenation, acute myocarditis

1. Introduction

Myocarditis is defined by the ESC as an inflammatory disease of the myocardium diagnosed by established histological, immunological and immunohistochemical criteria. Histological criteria consist of histological evidence of inflammatory infiltrates within the myocardium associated with myocyte degeneration and necrosis of non-ischemic origin while immunohistochemical criteria consist of ≥14 leucocytes/mm^2 including up to 4 monocytes/mm^2 with the presence of CD3 positive T-lymphocytes ≥7 cells/mm^2 [1].

IntechOpen

The clinical presentation of myocarditis varies significantly. It can range from acute coronary syndrome-like to acute or chronic heart failure forms. Specifically, it may present as acute chest pain frequently associated with recent infections, as new-onset heart failure (symptoms within 2 weeks to 3 months), as chronic heart failure (symptoms >3 months) or as a "life-threatening" – fulminant condition (refractory arrhythmias, cardiogenic shock). In general, acute coronary syndrome-like presentation has been associated with a better overall prognosis while heart failure is usually associated with a worse one, resulting in dilated cardiomyopathy or even death.

Diagnosis of acute myocarditis requires a workup consisting of both routine and specialized tests. ECG is usually abnormal in most cases, however, there are no specific signs. The most common findings are sinus tachycardia and repolarization abnormalities (either negative T waves or concave ST-T segment elevation as also seen in acute pericarditis) [1].

Unfortunately, there are no specific biomarkers for the diagnosis of myocarditis. Inflammatory markers are usually raised along with markers of myocardial injury (troponin, creatine kinase and its MB isoenzyme) and brain natriuretic peptides. Viral antibodies in the serum provide no information and may lead to an incorrect diagnosis. In general, only findings in myocardial tissue can be considered reliable with the exception of systemic diseases like hepatitis C, Lyme disease, HIV or rickettsial infections [1].

Echocardiography should always be performed in suspected myocarditis both for ruling out other cardiac diseases and for assessing ventricular function. In acute myocarditis, the findings may include regional wall motion abnormalities (usually beyond the supply area of coronary arteries), global ventricular dysfunction and/or pericardial effusion. Increased wall thickness may be observed most likely as a result of edema. Ventricular dilation is rare in the acute setting. While there are no specific signs seen through echocardiography, newer imaging techniques may provide some additional information since myocardial strain is most commonly affected in the inferolateral wall [2].

The exclusion of coronary artery disease should be performed in all patients suspected of myocarditis. This can be done through either classical or computed tomography coronary angiography.

The most important examination in myocarditis workup is the cardiac magnetic resonance (CMR) which provides information on both ventricular function and tissue characterization. In clinically stable patients, CMR can almost single-highhandedly confirm the diagnosis through the use of the updated Lake Louise criteria. These criteria require finding evidence of both myocardial edema (as seen through T2 mapping or T2-weighted images) and non-ischemic myocardial injury (as seen through T1 imaging, extracellular volume or late gadolinium enhancement) while supportive criteria include the presence of concomitant pericarditis or systolic left ventricular dysfunction [3]. For many years, the most commonly used criterion was the pattern of late gadolinium enhancement (LGE) which represent myocardial necrosis and fibrosis. In myocarditis, LGE is usually seen in the subepicardial and midmyocardial layers [4] and in the inferolateral wall [5]. Its presence in the anteroseptal wall is associated with a worse prognosis [6].

Despite the important role of CMR, diagnosis of myocarditis is confirmed through proposed criteria by a position statement of the European Society of Cardiology. A combination of at least 1 clinical and 1 para-clinical criteria is necessary or at least 2 para-clinical criteria in the case of asymptomatic patients. Clinical criteria include: (i) acute chest pain; (ii) new-onset or chronic heart failure symptoms; (iii) palpitation, unexplained arrhythmias or syncope and (iv) unexplained cardiogenic shock. Para-clinical criteria include: (i) ECG findings such as repolarization abnormalities, atrio-ventricular block, sinus tachycardia, frequent premature ventricular complexes etc.; (ii) elevated levels of troponin; (iii) functional and structural abnormalities on cardiac imaging and (iv) consistent findings through tissue characterization by CMR [1].

Treatment of myocarditis is consistent with heart failure treatment in hemodynamically stable patients. B-blockers and ACE inhibitors have been the mainstay of therapy for many decades with good results. The addition of mineralocorticoid receptor antagonists (MRAs) can be considered in cases of persistent left ventricular dysfunction. Newer treatments such as angiotensin receptor neprilysin inhibitors (ARNIs) or sodium-glucose co-transporter 2 inhibitors (SGLT2-i) have not been examined in myocarditis patients apart from animal studies [7, 8] but may prove useful in the future. Finally, device treatment such as ICD implantation is important in case of recurrent ventricular arrhythmias, aborted sudden cardiac death (as secondary prevention) or persistent ventricular dysfunction (as primary prevention). However, ICD implantation should be avoided in the acute setting, since arrhythmias may be ameliorated. In the above-mentioned cases of secondary prevention, wearable ICDs may be of use and the decision for permanent ICD implantation can take place during the follow-up [9]. More specialized myocarditis treatment (immunosuppressive treatment and mechanical circulatory support) will be further analyzed below.

This chapter will be mostly focused on fulminant variations since those generally have an indication for extracorporeal life support. Fulminant myocarditis requires urgent management and a quick referral to tertiary expert centers for advanced heart failure therapies. Due to its urgency, the diagnostic work-up should happen simultaneously with management. As a result, the first step usually includes imaging of the coronary arteries to exclude the possibility of the acute coronary syndrome. Management should include support of the respiratory system – usually requiring the use of either non-invasive or invasive ventilation – and circulatory support – requiring the use of inotropes or mechanical circulatory support in later stages [10].

While in less severe forms, diagnosis of myocarditis is often made through CMR, patients presenting with fulminant myocarditis are in a too critical condition to undergo this examination [11]. The "gold standard" for myocarditis diagnosis has long been the endomyocardial biopsy (EMB) which can also provide information on the specific etiology of myocarditis in each patient. From a pathological standpoint, there are three main types of myocarditis: lymphocytic, eosinophilic and giant-cell while, as far as etiology is of concern, it can be viral or non-viral. The differentiation of which type of myocarditis one deals with, is necessary for providing etiology-specific treatment. Specifically, viral forms of myocarditis may benefit from virus-specific treatment [12] (e.g. acyclovir for HHV-6, interferon for enteroviruses, etc.) while non-viral forms may benefit from immunosuppression. Eosinophilic myocarditis benefits from corticosteroid administration while also treating the underlying cause of eosinophilia (parasitic infections, hematologic syndromes, etc.). Finally, giant cell myocarditis is the variation with the worse prognosis requiring combination immunosuppressive treatment and consideration for urgent ventricular assist device implantation or heart transplantation [13–15]. As a result, it comes as no surprise that the performance of EMB in fulminant myocarditis patients is associated with a better prognosis [16, 17]. It should be noted that EMB may not necessarily reveal the proper etiology due to the absence of pathological findings from the sample site. In high clinical suspicion (especially in the case of giant-cell myocarditis), EMB should be repeated in order to acquire samples from different sites.

In cases where the patient's clinical condition rapidly deteriorates despite hemodynamic support, corticosteroids and even immunosuppression should be administered while awaiting biopsy results. Studies on both animal and human subjects have shown that corticosteroid administration has not been associated with exacerbation in the case of possible viral disease or worse overall prognosis in the case of fulminant myocarditis [18].

In critically ill patients with significantly reduced ejection fraction, inotrope administration may stabilize their clinical condition. However, the treating team should be ready to use mechanical circulatory support devices (intra-aortic balloon pump, percutaneous ventricular assist devices or extracorporeal membrane oxygenation).

2. Extracorporeal life support (ELS) or extracorporeal membrane oxygenation (ECMO)

Extracorporeal membrane oxygenation (ECMO) is a device that allows temporary support in pulmonary and/or cardiac failure refractory to conventional medical management [19]. It mainly consists of a blood pump, oxygenator, drainage and returns cannulae and arterial and venous access points (**Figure 1**). The blood pump propels the blood to the oxygenator membrane where the gas exchange between the patient's blood and the gas mixture of the device happens.

The ECMO has three main configurations depending on the access sites used: veno-venous (VV) ECMO, peripheral veno-arterial (VA) ECMO and central VA

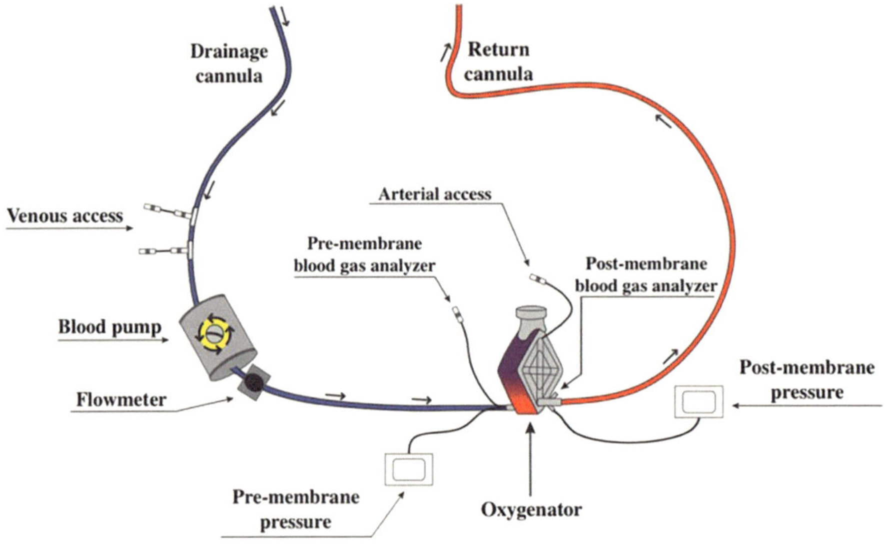

Figure 1.
A diagram demonstrating the components of an extracorporeal membrane oxygenation device [19]. (The figure is shared through the CC BY 4.0 according to the original article).

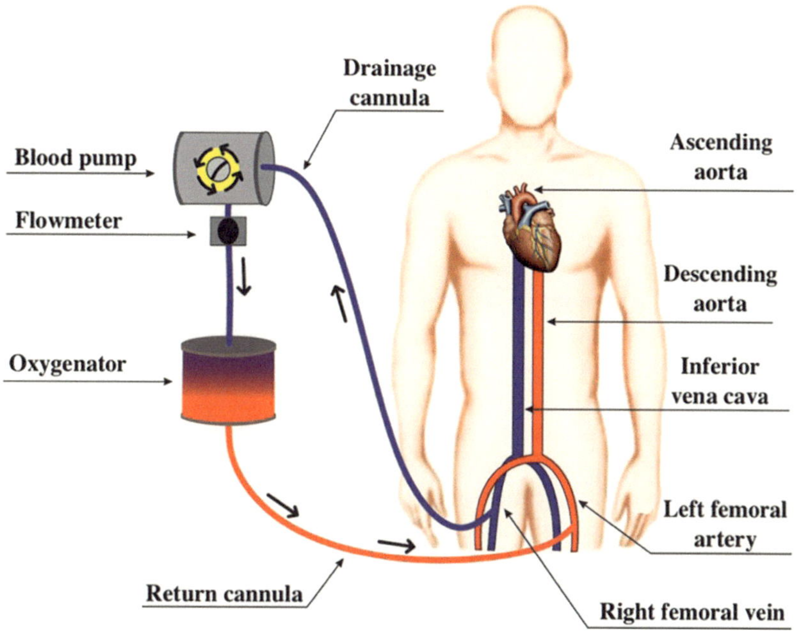

Figure 2.
A diagram demonstrating the most common peripheral VA ECMO configuration [19]. (The figure is shared through the CC BY 4.0 according to the original article).

ECMO. In VV ECMO, veins are used as both access sites with the purpose of supporting mainly the respiratory system. In this chapter, we will not focus on this configuration.

In VA ECMO, an artery and a vein are used as access sites. In central VA ECMO, the drainage cannula can be inserted directly into the right atrium, and the return cannula into the ascending aorta. On the other hand, in the peripheral VA ECMO, the drainage cannula is usually inserted into the femoral vein and the return cannula into the femoral artery (**Figure 2**). In this configuration, the patient's respiratory and circulatory systems are both supported essentially bypassing the heart and lungs providing oxygenated blood to peripheral organs. The heart still pumps blood up to the descending aorta depending on its systolic function.

The main complications of ECMO consist of device thrombosis, bleeding (access site, gastrointestinal or intracranial due to anticoagulation), acute kidney injury, limb ischemia (in peripheral configuration) and infection.

3. The role of extracorporeal membrane oxygenation in the management of acute myocarditis

Despite its complications, mechanical circulatory support is the most crucial and effective option in the management of fulminant myocarditis refractory to medical treatment providing valuable time for recovery either spontaneously or through the specific treatment described above.

Intra-aortic balloon pump (IABP) is usually the first option acting through afterload reduction and a small increase in cardiac output (around 0.5 L) [20]. Though its complication rate is relatively low compared to more invasive options, IABP cannot support worsening patients exactly due to its limitations of provided flow.

The next option is the percutaneous ventricular assist devices (pLVAD) which consist of Impella and TandemHeart – temporary LVADs implanted through the femoral artery. Their main advantage is the significant increase of cardiac output providing a flow of up to 5 L (depending on which model is used) along with a less invasive approach of surgically implanted VADs. Despite the small series of patients treated with this option, the reported results are generally satisfactory [21]. Their main disadvantages include the support of one ventricle only – usually the left one. As a consequence, this option is limited to patients with adequate right ventricular function to prevent the post-implantation development of right ventricular failure, unless two such devices are implanted simultaneously (one for each ventricle), thus, significantly increasing the odds of adverse effects.

Extracorporeal membrane oxygenation essentially bypasses the heart and provides adequate oxygenation to peripheral organs. Their main use in fulminant myocarditis is as bridge-to-recovery, bridge-to-transplant or bridge-to-bridge (bridge to a more permanent solution such as a durable VAD) in irreversible conditions often as a result of giant cell myocarditis. ECMO efficacy in fulminant myocarditis has been well described with survival rates of around 75% and VAD-free survival rates of around 61% [22, 23].

Even though ECMO supports the peripheral organs, it does not contribute to the unloading of the left ventricle. On the contrary, regardless of central or peripheral configuration, ECMO significantly increases the left ventricular afterload due to the retrograde flow to the aorta. In moderately reduced left ventricular systolic function with peripheral VA ECMO, this results in separate oxygenation of the upper and lower part of the body; the upper body is oxygenated by blood provided by the native flow through the heart while the lower body is oxygenated by blood provided by the device with the "splash" zone lying at some point in the descending aorta [24]. In cases of inadequate lung function, this phenomenon may cause the Harlequin syndrome characterized by hypoxia and cyanosis of the upper body and normal saturation and color of the lower body. The syndrome can be resolved by changing the configuration to a central one whereas the device provides oxygenated blood directly to the ascending aorta. This complication is rare when dealing with fulminant myocarditis due to the generally adequate lung function and the significantly reduced left ventricular function resulting in device blood supply to the whole body since the retrograde flow reaches the ascending aorta.

The above-described increased afterload combined with the significantly reduced ventricular function result in a perpetually loaded left ventricle potentially hindering recovery. In some cases, the aortic valve may remain closed during the cardiac cycle due to the inability of the cardiac muscle fibers to generate enough force/pressure to overcome the increased afterload. This phenomenon is nicely demonstrated by pressure-volume loops (PV loops) (**Figure 3**) which show a significant reduction of stroke volume with increasing ECMO flows. Potential solutions include the concurrent use of IABP, pVADs or direct transaortic left ventricular venting. All of these options provide some amount of left ventricular unloading thus promoting cardiac recovery [25].

Another main ECMO disadvantage is its temporary nature. In general, ECMO support cannot last the past 14 days due to a significant increase in adverse effects with prolonged support. Bleeding due to continuous heparin administration,

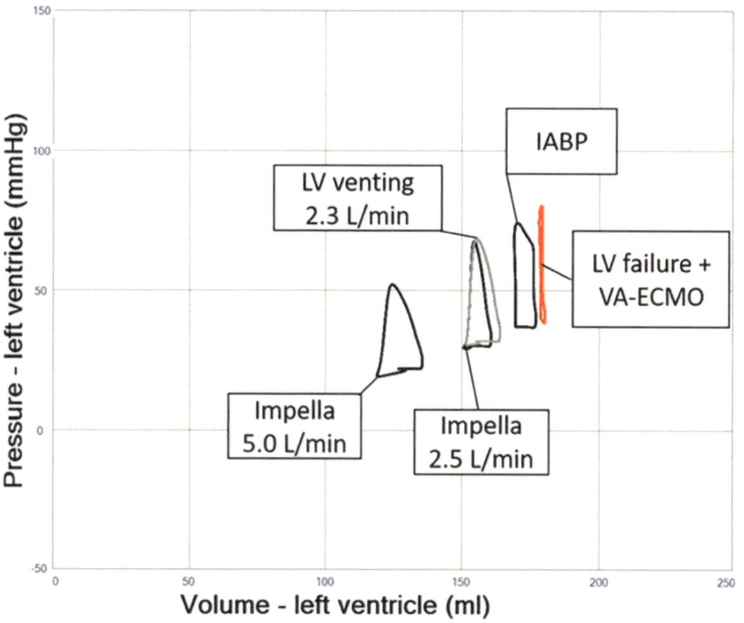

Figure 3.
A simulation showing the unloading potential of IABP, LV venting and Impella in a significantly deteriorated left ventricle supported with ECMO [25]. (The figure is shared through the CC BY 4.0 according to the original article).

infections and limb ischemia are common in these cases. Specifically for patients with myocarditis, it has been reported that prolonged ECMO support >7 days is associated with a worse prognosis [26]. However, this association could also be explained by the patients' worse clinical conditions resulting to prolonged ECMO support.

Reported predictors of myocarditis patient outcomes supported with ECMO include clinical characteristics, biomarkers and echocardiographic characteristics. The most important clinical predictor is the prolonged prevalence of arrhythmias be they atrioventricular block or ventricular arrhythmias [27]. SOFA score has also been associated with the patient outcome with scores >12 shown to be predictive of death or established heart failure [28]. CK-MB is the most well-reported biomarker with two independent studies agreeing to its prognostic value with levels >95 ng/mL [28] or > 185 IU/L [27] predicting a lower chance of successful weaning. Finally, the only echocardiographic parameter shown to have some prognostic value is the left ventricular posterior wall thickness with better results when >11 mm [27]. Unfortunately, all of the referenced studies are based on a small series due to the low incidence of myocarditis and even lower of its fulminant presentation.

4. Conclusion

Fulminant myocarditis is a rare yet significantly dangerous syndrome that needs urgent referral to tertiary centers for endomyocardial biopsy, advanced heart failure treatments and etiology-specific treatment. Mechanical circulatory support is the cornerstone of its management with extracorporeal membrane oxygenation devices being the last resort in conditions refractory to medical and less invasive mechanical circulatory support measures. The outcomes with ECMO devices are more than acceptable with a 75% survival rate especially when combined with solutions for adequate left ventricular unloading.

Author details

Aggeliki Gkouziouta
Onassis Cardiac Surgery Centre, Athens, Greece

*Address all correspondence to: agkouziouta@yahoo.gr

References

[1] Caforio ALP, Pankuweit S, Arbustini E, Basso C, Gimeno-Blanes J, Felix SB, et al. Current state of knowledge on aetiology, diagnosis, management, and therapy of myocarditis: A position statement of the European Society of Cardiology Working Group on Myocardial and Pericardial Diseases. European Heart Journal. 2013;**34**(33):2636, 2648a-2648, 2648d

[2] Meindl C, Paulus M, Poschenrieder F, Zeman F, Maier LS, Debl K. Patients with acute myocarditis and preserved systolic left ventricular function: Comparison of global and regional longitudinal strain imaging by echocardiography with quantification of late gadolinium enhancement by CMR. Clinical Research in Cardiology: Official Journal of the German Cardiac Society. 2021;**110**(11):1792-1800

[3] Ferreira VM, Schulz-Menger J, Holmvang G, Kramer CM, Carbone I, Sechtem U, et al. Cardiovascular magnetic resonance in nonischemic myocardial inflammation: Expert recommendations. Journal of the American College of Cardiology. 2018;**72**(24):3158-3176

[4] Valevičienė N, Petrulionienė Z, Petrauskienė B, Lauraitis G, Glaveckaitė S, Palionis D, et al. Differentiation of acute myocarditis and acute myocardial infarction by the regional distribution of myocardial irreversible injury using cardiovascular magnetic resonance imaging. Medicina (Kaunas, Lithuania). 2012;**48**(3):132-137

[5] Adamopoulos S, Miliopoulos D, Karavidas A, Nikolaou M, Lazaros G, Gkouziouta A, et al. Hellenic registry on myocarditis syndromes on behalf of hellenic heart failure association: The HERMES-HF Registry. ESC Heart Failure. 2020;7(6):3676-3684

[6] Aquaro GD, Perfetti M, Camastra G, Monti L, Dellegrottaglie S, Moro C, et al. Cardiac MR with late gadolinium enhancement in acute myocarditis with preserved systolic function: ITAMY study. Journal of the American College of Cardiology. 2017;**70**(16):1977-1987

[7] Liang W, Xie BK, Ding PW, Wang M, Yuan J, Cheng X, et al. Sacubitril/valsartan alleviates experimental autoimmune myocarditis by inhibiting Th17 cell differentiation independently of the NLRP3 inflammasome pathway. Frontiers in Pharmacology. 2021;**12**:727838

[8] Long Q, Li L, Yang H, Lu Y, Yang H, Zhu Y, et al. SGLT2 inhibitor, canagliflozin, ameliorates cardiac inflammation in experimental autoimmune myocarditis. International Immunopharmacology. 2022;**110**:109024

[9] Doz P, Sperzel J. Value of the wearable cardioverter defibrillator (WCD) as a bridging-therapy before implantation of a cardioverter defibrillator (ICD). Journal of Atrial Fibrillation. 2016;**8**(5):1247

[10] Hang W, Chen C, Seubert JM, Wang DW. Fulminant myocarditis: A comprehensive review from etiology to treatments and outcomes. Signal Transduction and Targeted Therapy. 2020;**5**(1):287

[11] Kociol RD, Cooper LT, Fang JC, Moslehi JJ, Pang PS, Sabe MA, et al. Recognition and initial management of fulminant myocarditis: A scientific statement from the american heart association. Circulation. 2020;**141**(6):e69-e92

[12] Sinagra G, Porcari A, Gentile P, Artico J, Fabris E, Bussani R, et al. Viral

presence-guided immunomodulation in lymphocytic myocarditis: An update. European Journal of Heart Failure. 2021;**23**(2):211-216

[13] Rosenstein ED, Zucker MJ, Kramer N. Giant cell myocarditis: Most fatal of autoimmune diseases. Seminars in Arthritis and Rheumatism. 2000;**30**(1):1-16

[14] Kandolin R, Lehtonen J, Salmenkivi K, Räisänen-Sokolowski A, Lommi J, Kupari M. Diagnosis, treatment, and outcome of giant-cell myocarditis in the era of combined immunosuppression. Circulation. Heart Failure. 2013;**6**(1):15-22

[15] Cooper LT, Hare JM, Tazelaar HD, Edwards WD, Starling RC, Deng MC, et al. Usefulness of immunosuppression for giant cell myocarditis. The American Journal of Cardiology. 2008;**102**(11):1535-1539

[16] Ammirati E, Cipriani M, Moro C, Raineri C, Pini D, Sormani P, et al. Clinical presentation and outcome in a contemporary cohort of patients with acute myocarditis. Circulation. 2018;**138**(11):1088-1099

[17] Kondo T, Okumura T, Shibata N, Imaizumi T, Dohi K, Izawa H, et al. Differences in prognosis and cardiac function according to required percutaneous mechanical circulatory support and histological findings in patients with fulminant myocarditis: Insights from the change PUMP 2 study. Journal of the American Heart Association. 2022;**11**(4):e023719

[18] Li S, Xu S, Li C, Ran X, Cui G, He M, et al. A life support-based comprehensive treatment regimen dramatically lowers the in-hospital mortality of patients with fulminant myocarditis: A multiple center study. Science China. Life Sciences. 2019;**62**(3):369-380

[19] de RCF C, Rabello Filho R, Timenetsky KT, Moreira FT, da LCS V, de Bravim BA, et al. Extracorporeal membrane oxygenation: A literature review. Revista Brasileira de Terapia Intensiva. 2019;**31**(3):410-424

[20] Li H, Li L. Successful treatment of fulminant myocarditis with intra-aortic balloon pump counterpulsation combined with immunoglobulin and glucocorticoid in a young male adult. Frontiers in Cardiovascular Medicine. 2022;**9**:905189

[21] Annamalai SK, Esposito ML, Jorde L, Schreiber T, Hall AS, O'Neill WW, et al. The impella microaxial flow catheter is safe and effective for treatment of myocarditis complicated by cardiogenic shock: An analysis from the global cVAD registry. Journal of Cardiac Failure. 2018;**24**(10):706-710

[22] Tadokoro N, Fukushima S, Minami K, Taguchi T, Saito T, Kawamoto N, et al. Efficacy of central extracorporeal life support for patients with fulminant myocarditis and cardiogenic shock. European Journal of Cardio-thoracic Surgery: Official Journal of the European Association for Cardio-thoracic Surgery. 2021;**60**(5):1184-1192

[23] Cheng R, Hachamovitch R, Kittleson M, Patel J, Arabia F, Moriguchi J, et al. Clinical outcomes in fulminant myocarditis requiring extracorporeal membrane oxygenation: A weighted meta-analysis of 170 patients. Journal of Cardiac Failure. 2014;**20**(6):400-406

[24] Pasrija C, Bedeir K, Jeudy J, Kon ZN. Harlequin syndrome during venoarterial extracorporeal membrane oxygenation. Radiol Cardiothorac Imaging. 2019;**1**(2):e190031

[25] Donker DW, Brodie D, Henriques JPS, Broomé M. Left ventricular unloading during veno-arterial ECMO: A simulation study. ASAIO journal (American Society for Artificial Internal Organs : 1992). 2019;**65**(1):11-20

[26] Diddle JW, Almodovar MC, Rajagopal SK, Rycus PT, Thiagarajan RR. Extracorporeal membrane oxygenation for the support of adults with acute myocarditis. Critical Care Medicine. 2015;**43**(5):1016-1025

[27] Matsumoto M, Asaumi Y, Nakamura Y, Nakatani T, Nagai T, Kanaya T, et al. Clinical determinants of successful weaning from extracorporeal membrane oxygenation in patients with fulminant myocarditis. ESC Heart Failure. 2018;**5**(4):675-684

[28] Lee YI, Chung S, Yang JH, Sung K, Kim D, Choi JO, et al. Extracorporeal membrane oxygenation for fulminant myocarditis: Increase of cardiac enzyme and SOFA score is associated with high mortality. Journal of Clinical Medicine. 2021;**10**(7):1526

Chapter 4

ECMO as Bridge to Heart Transplantation

Andrea Lechiancole, Massimo Maiani, Igor Vendramin, Sandro Sponga and Ugolino Livi

Abstract

Extracorporeal membrane oxygenation (ECMO) is increasingly employed to support patients affected by refractory cardiogenic shock. When patients cannot be weaned from ECMO because of severe heart dysfunction, heart transplantation (HTx) or implantation of a durable mechanical circulatory support should be considered. Traditionally, the use of ECMO as a direct bridge to HTx was burdened by high mortality. However, during these last years, the widespread employment of ECMO increased centers' experience in the management of this device, and new allocation policies provided the highest priority level for ECMO HTx candidates. Therefore, these factors could have mitigated the negative outcomes previously reported. The aim of this chapter is to describe the role of ECMO as a direct bridge to HTx, analyzing results of this strategy, and how to determine candidacy and risk stratification among the severely ill population of patients supported by this mechanical circulatory support.

Keywords: ECMO, heart transplantation, bridge, cardiogenic shock, candidacy

1. Introduction

Venoarterial extracorporeal membrane oxygenation (ECMO) is a short-term mechanical circulatory support (MCS) that enables cardiopulmonary support. Thanks to the easily reproducible technique of implantation and its biventricular and respiratory support, ECMO can be deployed in a relatively short time in almost all cardiopulmonary failures. For this reason, it is a well-accepted therapeutic option for patients with refractory cardiogenic shock [1, 2].

Like all temporary MCS, ECMO is generally employed as a bridge to decision treatment [3]. The possible clinical scenarios after ECMO support are represented by: 1—weaning from the device secondary to the recovery of cardiac function, 2—bridge to a durable MCS (left or biventricular assist devices) or bridge to heart transplantation (HTx), or 3—ECMO discontinuation because of irreversible multiorgan failure.

Patients supported by ECMO have traditionally been considered as high-risk candidates for HTx, with the poor outcome on the waiting list and after transplantation [3–7]. Many institutions advocates favoring the bridge to a durable left ventricular assist device (LVAD) if the function of the right ventricle improves during

ECMO support. This strategy was largely adopted in the United States, aiming to consider HTx after the complete recovery of patient clinical conditions [8, 9]. However, the results of this so-called "double bridge to HTx" are controversial [9].

The United Network for Organ Sharing (UNOS) has recently changed the heart allocation policy and conferred the highest priority status to patients supported by ECMO [10], in line with other transplant organizations [11]. Therefore, the number of patients that cannot be weaned from ECMO support and are considered for direct heart transplantation (HTx) is increasing.

1.1 Candidacy for HTx in patients supported with ECMO

Bridging to a durable mechanical circulatory support or HTx is considered when patients could not be weaned from the ECMO support because of a missed recovery of the myocardial function. Several weaning protocols are described in the literature [12, 13] and almost universally consist in the gradual reduction of the ECMO support, while hemodynamics and echocardiography parameters are monitored. If the cardiac function is deemed severely and irreversibly impaired, a rapid assessment of the patient clinical conditions should be performed before listing for HTx.

The first step when considering a candidacy for HTx is the evaluation of neurological function since de-novo disabling cerebrovascular accidents generally prevent patients from being listed. Severe neurological complications could occur as a consequence of cardiogenic shock, particularly after cardiac arrest and cardiopulmonary resuscitation, or during cannulation and duration of ECMO support. However, severe hypoperfusion and prolonged immobilization could result in critical illness with severe impairment of musculoskeletal function. A thorough examination is essential to discriminate between this potentially reversible condition to others. Cerebral imaging, usually by means of computed tomography (CT), is usually performed to exclude acute cerebrovascular accidents (strokes or hemorrhages) or neoplasms.

Patients already on the waitlist for HTx at the time of ECMO implantation generally do not need any additional diagnostic exams. However, patients who are evaluated for HTx candidacy, while on ECMO support, are generally screened by means of a whole-body CT scan, and also all pathological conditions should be assessed. In fact, persistent end-organ dysfunction, while on ECMO support, has been strongly associated with poor prognosis after HTx [14–16]. Lastly, when considering patient age limits, they could vary according to clinical status, but generally an age > 70 years preclude an HTx eligibility (**Figure 1**).

1.2 ECMO as BTT management

Once weaning attempts have confirmed an irreversible severe heart impairment, the ultimate goal of ECMO support is to permit adequate perfusion for end-organ recovery.

Typically, venoarterial ECMO is effective in reducing the right atrial pressure and in increasing the mean arterial blood pressure. The systemic arterio-venous pressure gradient is fundamental in enhancing tissue of organs with portal circulation, such as the liver and kidney. Thus, a relatively high ECMO-generated blood flow is of paramount importance to allow end-organ function improvement.

However, the major risk of this strategy is left ventricular overdistension. In fact, the failing left ventricle (LV) contraction could not be able to generate an adequate

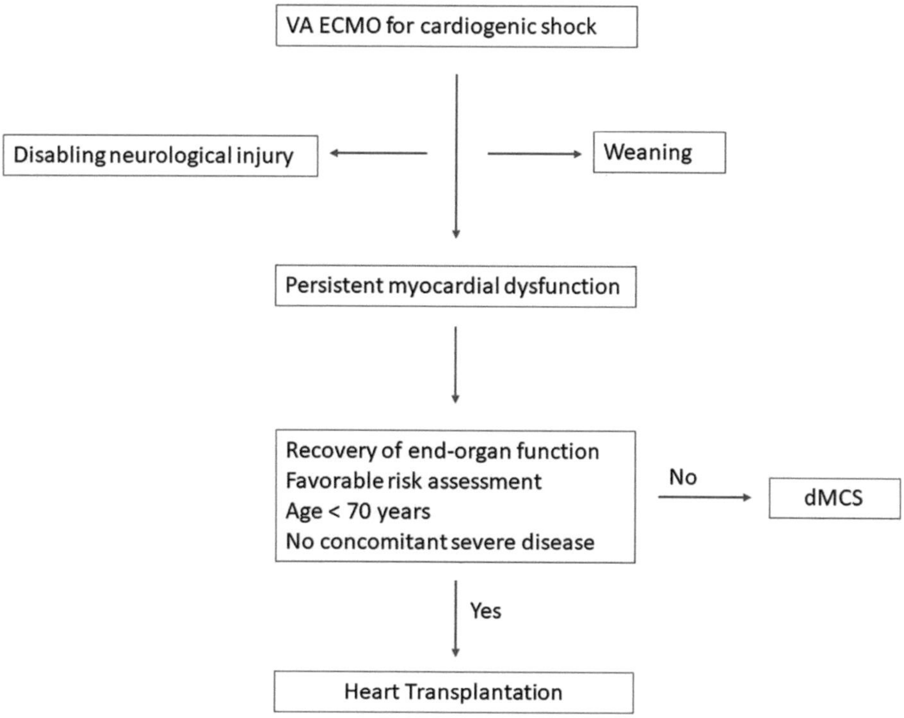

Figure 1.
Proposed decisional algorithm for patients supported by ECMO. VA ECMO: venoarterial extracorporeal membrane oxygenation and dMCS: durable mechanical circulatory support.

pressure to overcome the ECMO-derived afterload, and at the end to open the aortic valve. This condition could hesitate to blood stasis within the LV, with increased pressure inside the chamber and eventually pulmonary edema. Chest radiography and echo imaging are useful in promptly recognizing and monitoring these conditions and sequelae. However, the employment of a pulmonary artery catheter represents the most direct and time-sensitive means of detecting LV loading and permits to measure the pulmonary capillary wedge pressure (PCWP) and pulmonary artery pressure.

Once there is evidence of elevated PCWP or LV overdistension and pulmonary edema, a LV venting strategy should be introduced. It is worth of note that many centers employed a LV unloading strategy in an early phase of the ECMO course to prevent or limit as most as possible pulmonary congestion, while assuring adequate blood flow and pressure in the systemic circulation.

There are different strategies described for LV unloading, and clinical practice is generally guided by local expertise and experience. A combination of reduction of ECMO flow, vasodilators, and inotropes could facilitate the opening of the aortic valve, but peripheral perfusion could be compromised and noneffective in assure end-organ recovery.

Intra-aortic balloon pump (IABP) is the most widely used ancillary invasive support. It could be deployed at the bedside and generally with no difficulties. IABP reduces blood pressure into the aortic root during systole, enhancing aortic valve opening and LV ejection. However, IABP is effective in LV unloading only when some residual contractility of the LV is present, and its role in affecting outcomes among patients supported by ECMO is still not clarified [17].

Direct LV venting could be accomplished by means of a cannula surgically placed into the LV and connected to the venous line of the ECMO circuit or through the deployment of the impella (abiomed, danvers, and MA), a percutaneous transaortic ventricular assist device that provides an antegrade micro-axial flow. The ECPELLA strategy (ECMO + Impella) has emerged as an attractive solution since it combines the positive effect of high-flow arterial support with an efficient LV unloading [18]. A certain level of expertise and technical skills are the main limitation of direct LV venting strategies, that are generally offered in facilities specialized in ECMO support.

1.3 Outcomes of BTT with ECMO

The scientific evidence about the use of VA ECMO as a bridge to HTx is limited, and most studies are single-center or based on the analysis of the UNOS registry.

Despite the improvement of ECMO technology and increased experience in managing supported patients, HTx bridged by ECMO continues to be suboptimal when compared to patients bridged with left ventricular assist devices (LVAD) or without the need of MCS, and still burdened by significant mortality. In fact, 1 year after HTX, the overall survival rate for this group of patients is reported to be 60–70% [5, 6]. In particular, survival probability decreases abruptly within the first 30 days after HTx, when the mortality rate is reported as high as 20–40%. Multiorgan failure, primary graft failure, and sepsis account for a great part of early deaths [4–6].

Since the main limitation of HTx is the shortage of the donor pool, an accurate risk stratification among HTx candidates on ECMO support could limit as most as possible any shifting of available organs avoiding futile treatments. The severe hypoperfusion that accompanies cardiogenic shock affects the function of end-organs, by means of metabolic alterations at the cellular and extracellular levels whose severity is strictly related to the duration and degree of hypoperfusion, and to baseline pathological alterations.

It has been reported that persistent or worsening end-organ failure is strongly related to poor outcomes after HTX. Renal failure and mechanical ventilation were strong predictors of mortality according to Zalawadiya et al. [14], who analyzed the UNOS registry to report the outcomes of BTT with VA ECMO from 2000 to 2015.

Jansseron et al. [11] and Coutance et al. [16] further confirm the negative role of renal impairment on survival after BTT with ECMO. According to the France experience, patients with a glomerular filtration rate < 40 mg/dl or in renal replacement treatment are no longer considered as HTx candidates. Moreover, patients are recommended to be awakened and extubated during ECMO support in order to prevent pulmonary complications related to prolonged mechanical ventilation.

Other conditions that were reported to be risk factors for death are infection, high levels of lactate, and liver dysfunction [5, 6–19].

Scoring systems have been advocated by some authors for risk assessment, since they permit to stratify clinical status of patients in an objective and reproducible way, taking into account several clinical variables. Since they permit to comprehensively consider different clinical and biochemical values, risk scores could be considered as a surrogate of disease, and have proved to effectively predict survival in HTx bridged with ECMO.

In a previous study of our group, the acutephysiology, age, and chronic health evaluation (APACHE) IV score was demonstrated to be a powerful predictor of survival, with a receiving operative curve of 0.98. In particular, patients with an APACHE IV score > 47, 30 days and 1 year survival were 40% and 26.6%, respectively, significantly higher than the group with an APACHE IV score < 47 (30 days and 1 year survival of 100% and 89.7%, respectively) [20].

The alternative scoring system effectively employed in risk stratification among BTT with ECMO were sequential organ failure assessment (SOFA) and the model for end-stage liver disease excluding international normalize ratio (MELD-XI) [7, 21].

Large multicentric prospective studies are necessary to determine the accuracy and efficacy of these risk scores, and cut-off values that could discriminate between favorable or poor outcomes.

1.4 Listing ECMO patients

Since patients supported with ECMO have the highest risk for mortality on the transplant waitlist, they were given a preferential status at listing in many countries. Since October 2018 even in the United States BTT with ECMO reached the highest priority status, and the number of patients who are being bridged to HT with ECMO is constantly increasing [8]. As reported in a recent analysis using the UNOS database, the introduction of the new allocation system enhanced the access to available organs for HTx candidates supported with ECMO, resulting in a higher rate of HTx with lower time on the waiting list [10]. Moreover, the post-HTx survival of ECMO-bridged recipients significantly improved, reaching 90% at months [10]. A similar survival result, 85% at one post-HTx year, was reported by a French group after the introduction of the new national French allocation protocol, that conferred the highest priority status for ECMO-supported patients and excluded for HTx patients with severely impaired renal function [16].

An alternative possible explanation for improved post-transplant survival of ECMO-supported patients with the new allocations systems could be related to the utilization of ECMO on a different cohort of patients. In fact, since patients supported with ECMO have a high likelihood of being transplanted, ECMO could be increasingly considered as the short-term MCS of choice to bridge patients.

On the other hand, patients supported with ECMO who could not be weaned and have major risk factors may warrant consideration for an alternative to HT, such as LVAD implantation. In fact, it has been argued that perhaps a strategy of transitioning ECMO supported patients to durable MCS may provide the stabilization required to guarantee better post HT outcomes and more judicious use of transplanted hearts [9, 19], but limited and controversial evidence does not permit to generate recommendations.

2. Udine experience

Out of 410 Htx performed at the University Hospital of Udine since 2005, a total of 41 (10%) patients were directly bridged to HTx with ECMO. The ECMO circuit consisted of a centrifugal blood pump (Rotaflow, Maquet, Hirrlingen, Germany) with a hollow fiber oxygenator (Quadrox). Tubes (33 mL of priming), as well as the oxygenator and the pump, were coated with bioline (maquet), which combines polypeptides and heparin.

Clinical characteristics of the population at the time of HTx are shown in **Table 1**. In brief, the median age was 57 years (range 38–73 years), and 80% (n = 33) were male patients. The median creatinine level was 1.6 mg/dl (range 0.8–3.5 mg/dl), and the rate of renal replacement treatment was 15% (n = 6). 25 patients (61%) were mechanically

	Overall population (n = 41)	Low-risk (n = 30)	High-risk (n = 11)	P
Median age (range), years	57 (38–73)	56 (38–69)	58 (41–73)	0.2
Male sex, n (%)	33 (80)	24 (80)	9 (82)	0.9
Median creatinine (range), mg/dl	1.6 (0.8–3.5)	1.6 (0.8–2.3)	1.7 (0.8–3.5)	0.5
Hemodialysis, n (%)	6 (15)	3 (10)	3 (27)	0.2
IABP, n (%)	32 (78)	23 (77)	9 (82)	0.8
Impella, n (%)	2 (5)	2 (7)	0 (0)	0.6
Mechanical ventilation, n (%)	25 (61)	15 (50)	10 (91)	0.02
Median duration of ECMO support (range), days	10 (3–21)	11 (5–21)	9 (2–19)	0.9
Donor age	47 (21–63)	46 (29–58)	49 (21–63)	0.2
Median ischemic graft time (range), minutes	210 (145–290)	220 (155–290)	200 (145–250)	0.3

Table 1.
Baseline clinical characteristics of patients bridged to HTx with ECMO support.

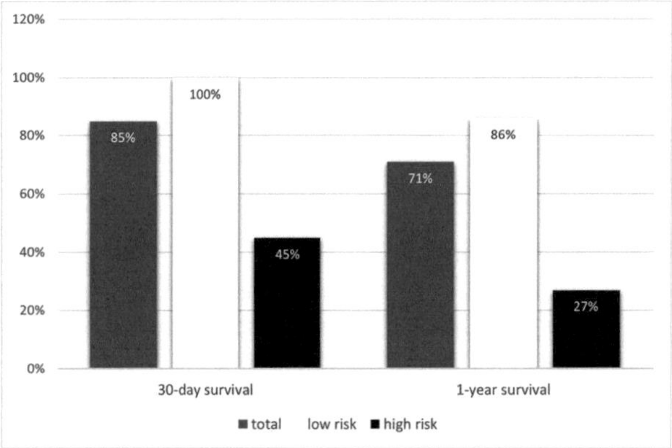

Figure 2.
Survival at 30 days and at 1 year of the overall population (total), APACHE IV score < 47 population (low-risk) and APACHE IV score ≥ 47 population (high-risk).

ventilated, 32 (78%) had IABP, and 2 (5%) an impella support for LV unloading. The median duration of ECMO support was 10 days (range 3–21 days).

After HTx, 30 days mortality was 15% (n = 6), and 1 year survival was 71% (six patients died after a median time from HTx of 73 days, range 42–237 days).

Since our previous experience revealed very poor outcomes for patients with values of APACHE IV score ≥ 47 [], we further extensively adopted this tool to stratify patients into two groups: low-risk (if APACHE IV score value was <47) and high-risk (APACHE IV score ≥ 47).

The low-risk group (n = 30) and the high-risk group (n = 11) had a median APACHE IV score of 34 (range 28–45) and 52 (47–60), respectively ($p < 0.001$).

As shown in the **Figure 2**, compared to other patients, those having an APACHE IV score had a significantly lower 30 days survival ($p < 0.001$) and 1 year-survival ($p < 0.001$).

3. Conclusions

VA ECMO as a BTT strategy is increasingly used after the change of allocation policies in many countries, particularly in the United States. Indeed, since patients supported with ECMO receive the highest priority status, this MCS has emerged as an attractive therapy to obtain at the same time cardiopulmonary support and to facilitate HTx.

However, since the ECMO-BTT strategy was traditionally burdened by high mortality, preventing any possible shifts of the limited available donor organ pool represents a major concern. Based on international experience, the key factors for obtaining successful HTx in patients supported with ECMO are as follows: 1—a thorough ECMO management aimed to prevent possible complications, while permitting end-organ recovery, 2—risk stratification and accurate selection of candidates at the time of listing, and 3—obtaining a compatible donor heart in relatively short time.

Otherwise, in high-risk conditions, transition to durable MCS should be considered to favor patient full recovery, permitting a judicious use of the limited donor pool.

Conflict of interest

The authors have no conflicts to declare.

Author details

Andrea Lechiancole*, Massimo Maiani, Igor Vendramin, Sandro Sponga and Ugolino Livi
Cardiothoracic Department, University Hospital of Udine, Italy

*Address all correspondence to: andrea.lechiancole@asufc.sanita.fvg.it

References

[1] Keebler ME, Haddad EV, Choi CW, McGrane S, Zalawadiya S, Schlendorf KH, et al. Venoarterial extracorporeal membrane oxygenation in cardiogenic shock. JACC: Heart Failure. 2018;**6**(6):503-516. DOI: 10.1016/j.jchf.2017.11.017

[2] Tsangaris A, Alexy T, Kalra R, Kosmopoulos M, Elliott A, Bartos JA, et al. Overview of veno-arterial extracorporeal membrane oxygenation (VA-ECMO) support for the management of cardiogenic shock. Frontiers in Cardiovascular Medicine. 2021;**7**(8):686558. DOI: 10.3389/fcvm.2021.686558

[3] Rousse N, Juthier F, Pinçon C, Hysi I, Banfi C, Robin E, et al. ECMO as a bridge to decision: Recovery, VAD, or heart transplantation? International Journal of Cardiology. 2015;**187**:620-627. DOI: 10.1016/j.ijcard.2015.03.283. Epub 2015 Mar 20

[4] Moonsamy P, Axtell AL, Ibrahim NE, Funamoto M, Tolis G, Lewis GD, et al. Survival after heart transplantation in patients bridged with mechanical circulatory support. Journal of the American College of Cardiology. 2020;**75**(23):2892-2905. DOI: 10.1016/j.jacc.2020.04.037

[5] Urban M, Siddique A, Merritt-Genore H, Um J. What are the results of venoarterial extracorporeal membrane oxygenation bridging to heart transplantation? Interactive Cardiovascular and Thoracic Surgery. 2019;**29**(4):632-634. DOI: 10.1093/icvts/ivz096

[6] Montisci A, Donatelli F, Cirri S, Coscioni E, Maiello C, Napoli C. Veno-arterial extracorporeal membrane oxygenation as bridge to heart transplantation: The way forward. Transplantation direct. 2021;**7**(8):e720. DOI: 10.1097/TXD.0000000000001172

[7] Fukuhara S, Takeda K, Kurlansky PA, Naka Y, Takayama H. Extracorporeal membrane oxygenation as a direct bridge to heart transplantation in adults. The Journal of Thoracic and Cardiovascular Surgery. 2018;**155**(4):1607-1618.e6. DOI: 10.1016/j.jtcvs.2017.10.152

[8] DeFilippis EM, Clerkin K, Truby LK, Francke M, Fried J, Masoumi A, et al. ECMO as a bridge to left ventricular assist device or heart transplantation. JACC Heart Failure. 2021;**9**(4):281-289. DOI: 10.1016/j.jchf.2020.12.012

[9] Coeckelenbergh S, Valente F, Mortier J, Engelman E, Roussoulières A, El Oumeiri B, et al. Long-term outcome after venoarterial extracorporeal membrane oxygenation as bridge to left ventricular assist device preceding heart transplantation. Journal of Cardiothoracic and Vascular Anesthesia. 2022;**36**(6):1694-1702. DOI: 10.1053/j.jvca.2021.06.035

[10] Gonzalez MH, Acharya D, Lee S, Leacche M, Boeve T, Manandhar-Shrestha N, et al. Improved survival after heart transplantation in patients bridged with extracorporeal membrane oxygenation in the new allocation system. The Journal of Heart and Lung Transplantation. 2021;**40**(2):149-157. DOI: 10.1016/j.healun.2020.11.004

[11] Jasseron C, Lebreton G, Cantrelle C, Legeai C, Leprince P, Flecher E, et al. Impact of heart transplantation on survival in patients on venoarterial extracorporeal membrane oxygenation

at listing in France. Transplantation. 2016;**100**(9):1979-1987. DOI: 10.1097/TP.0000000000001265

[12] Vuthoori R, Heaney C, Lima B, Knisel A, Miller E, Kennedy K, et al. Assessment of cardiac recovery in patients supported with venoarterial extracorporeal membrane oxygenation. ESC Heart Failure. 22 Apr 2022. DOI: 10.1002/ehf2.13892

[13] Trahanas JM, Li SS, Crowley JC, Ton VK, Funamoto M, Cudemus Deseda GA, et al. How to turn it down: The evidence and opinions behind adult venoarterial extracorporeal membrane oxygenation weaning. ASAIO Journal. 2021;**67**(9):964-972. DOI: 10.1097/MAT.0000000000001375

[14] Zalawadiya S, Fudim M, Bhat G, Cotts W, Lindenfeld J. Extracorporeal membrane oxygenation support and post-heart transplant outcomes among United States adults. The Journal of Heart and Lung Transplantation. 2017;**36**(1):77-81. DOI: 10.1016/j.healun.2016.10.008. Epub 2016 Oct 15

[15] Ivey-Miranda JB, Maulion C, Farrero-Torres M, Griffin M, Posada-Martinez EL, Testani JM, et al. Risk stratification of patients listed for heart transplantation while supported with extracorporeal membrane oxygenation. The Journal of Thoracic and Cardiovascular Surgery. 2021;**S0022-5223**(21):00877-00871. DOI: 10.1016/j.jtcvs.2021.05.032

[16] Coutance G, Jacob N, Demondion P, Nguyen LS, Bouglé A, Bréchot N, et al. Favorable outcomes of a direct heart transplantation strategy in selected patients on extracorporeal membrane oxygenation support. Critical Care Medicine. 2020;**48**(4):498-506. DOI: 10.1097/CCM.0000000000004182

[17] Barge-Caballero G, Castel-Lavilla MA, Almenar-Bonet L, Garrido-Bravo IP, Delgado JF, Rangel-Sousa D, et al. Venoarterial extracorporeal membrane oxygenation with or without simultaneous intra-aortic balloon pump support as a direct bridge to heart transplantation: Results from a nationwide Spanish registry. Interactive Cardiovascular and Thoracic Surgery. 2019;**29**(5):670-677. DOI: 10.1093/icvts/ivz155

[18] Meani P, Lorusso R, Pappalardo F. ECPella: Concept, physiology and clinical applications. Journal of Cardiothoracic and Vascular Anesthesia. 2022;**36**(2):557-566. DOI: 10.1053/j.jvca.2021.01.056

[19] Sponga S, Nagpal AD, Vendramin I, Ferrara V, Lechiancole A, Maiani M, et al. Bridge to heart transplantation in patients with cardiogenic shock: A 20-year experience with two different surgical strategies. Journal of Cardiovascular Medicine (Hagerstown, Md.). 2021;**22**(5):388-395. DOI: 10.2459/JCM.0000000000001097

[20] Lechiancole A, Sponga S, Isola M, Vendramin I, Maiani M, Livi U. Heart transplantation in patients supported by ECMO: Is the APACHE IV score a predictor of survival? Artificial Organs. 2018;**42**(6):670-673. DOI: 10.1111/aor.13099

[21] Chung JC, Tsai PR, Chou NK, Chi NH, Wang SS, Ko WJ. Extracorporeal membrane oxygenation bridge to adult heart transplantation. Clinical Transplantation. 2010;**24**(3):375-380. DOI: 10.1111/j.1399-0012.2009.01084.x

Chapter 5

The Role of Extracorporeal Membrane Oxygenation Support after Pulmonary Thrombo-Endarterectomy

Antonio Loforte, Gregorio Gliozzi, Giulio Giovanni Cavalli, Carlo Mariani, Luca Botta, Nazzareno Galiè, Davide Pacini and Sofia Martin-Suarez

Abstract

Chronic thromboembolic pulmonary hypertension (CTEPH) is a rare consequence of acute or chronic pulmonary embolism. Pulmonary endarterectomy (PEA) is the gold standard treatment: expert centers are able to offer this challenging procedure with low in-hospital mortality, excellent hemodynamic results, and significant improvement in exercise tolerance and quality of life. Despite careful preoperative selection and increasing technical experience in PEA, some patients may suffer from life-threatening complications requiring extracorporeal life support (ECLS). ECLS is necessary in case of heart failure, respiratory failure, or both. According to different indications and timing, cardiopulmonary failure after PEA should be managed with a tailored approach: veno-venous or veno-arterial support, and central or peripheral cannulation. In the present chapter, causes, management strategies, and outcomes of perioperative ECLS for PEA are discussed.

Keywords: extracorporeal life support (ECLS), pulmonary endarterectomy (PEA), chronic thromboembolic pulmonary hypertension (CTEPH), surgical strategies, outcomes of perioperative ECLS

1. Introduction

Chronic thromboembolic pulmonary hypertension (CTEPH) is a rare consequence of acute or chronic pulmonary embolism (PE). It has been estimated that it occurs in about 3% of acute PE survivors [1]. CTEPH has unique pathogenesis and a potentially curative surgical treatment other than pulmonary transplantation: for these reasons it represents the 4th group of pulmonary hypertensions (PH), according to the Nice classification [2]. CTEPH has been defined as "dual compartments vascular disease" because the occlusive disease due to fibrotic organization of thromboembolic lesions is associated with arterial wall hypertrophy and vasospasm of non-occluded segments, which leads to progressive development of PH and to right ventricular (RV) dysfunction [3–5]. Diagnosis and clinical management of CTEPH requires a dedicated multidisciplinary high-skilled team that could offer the entire range of therapeutical options: from medical therapy to balloon pulmonary angioplasty (BPA) and pulmonary endarterectomy (PEA) [6]. PEA is the treatment of choice in CTEPH [7]: technically, the operation is performed through full median sternotomy, cardiopulmonary bypass, myocardial arrest and myocardial protection, intermittent deep hypothermic circulatory arrest (DHCA). Patients should be carefully selected in order to balance surgical risk and optimal outcomes. Preoperative anatomical and hemodynamic information are crucial for preoperative risk stratification and surgical feasibility assessment. Nowadays, expert centers are able to offer this challenging procedure with low in-hospital mortality (<5%), excellent hemodynamic results, and significant improvement in exercise tolerance and quality of life [8].

Nevertheless, despite careful selection, some patients may suffer from life-threatening perioperative cardiorespiratory decompensation requiring extracorporeal life support (ECLS): in the present chapter, we are going to discuss causes, management strategies, and outcomes of perioperative ECLS for PEA.

2. Perioperative role and indications of ECLS in PEA

The mechanism of PH in CTEPH is multifactorial: the first step is due to the fibrotic organization of acute emboli that chronically occlude proximal pulmonary arteries (main, lobar, and segmental), the second step is the redistribution of blood flow and increase of shear stress in nonoccluded segments. Then micro-vasculopathy (affecting muscular pulmonary arteries, capillaries, and veins) progressively induces the increase in PVR, onset of symptoms, and, at last, RV dysfunction and failure [4, 5].

Timely diagnosis and treatment prevent from worsening of PH and reduce perioperative morbidity and mortality because a more compromised hemodynamic status is at higher risk of perioperative need for ECLS [9].

Basically, there are three main indications for ECLS:

- pure respiratory failure defined as hypoxia with pulse oximetry oxygen saturation (SO_2) less than 90% despite mechanical ventilation with 100% fraction of inspired oxygen (FiO_2), without preexisting hemodynamic failure;

- pure hemodynamic failure defined as circulatory failure precluding weaning from CPB or new-onset cardiogenic shock requiring maximal inotropic, without prior respiratory failure;

- mixed respiratory and hemodynamic failure defined as any combination of signs of both respiratory and hemodynamic failure [9–11].

Patients could require ECLS with three different therapeutical approaches or strategies:

- Bridge to surgery: the target is hemodynamic stabilization in patients with preoperative acute severe cardiorespiratory decompensation;

- Bridge to recovery (BTR): post-cardiotomy mechanical support if weaning from CPB is not possible or in case of organ failure in intensive care unit;

- Bridge to transplantation (BTT): in case of impossible weaning from ECLS in patients eligible for lung or heart-lung transplantation [9, 11].

The vast majority of patients are referred in stable conditions with long-standing symptoms but, in a few cases, such as in acute-on-chronic PE or massive main trunk involvement, patients could rapidly deteriorate with respiratory failure and/or cardiogenic shock due to RV failure: in these cases, PEA should not be further deferred, but ECLS could be the only chance of preoperative stabilization, especially in non-expert centers, allowing urgent PEA as next step [9, 12].

In stable patients, an appropriate preoperative evaluation allows the risk stratification of postoperative heart and lung failure: many clinical features may represent a red flag, and surgeons should forecast and plan the appropriate strategy, including ECLS and, even, organ transplantation [9, 11].

The anatomical location of thromboembolic lesions, assessed with multimodal imaging, is extremely important: distal lesions are not a contraindication, but they make surgery technically demanding, also in expert hands. High PVR increases the risk of an unsuccessful procedure and persistent residual PH, especially in case of unfavorable anatomy [9, 13].

However, distal lesions and high PVR alone must not be considered formal contraindications for surgery. In many series, patients with a need for ECLS often demonstrated preoperative high PVR and previous signs and symptoms of RV failure [9, 11, 13–15].

Regardless of the preoperative clinical profile, PEA patients are prone to specific severe complications tightly linked to surgical trauma, such as reperfusion edema/injury, bronchial or parenchymal bleeding, residual pulmonary hypertension, and RV failure.

As originally described by Jamieson, PEA consists of a "true endarterectomy": the surgeon must identify a subintimal cleavage plane in order to be radical, removing entirely the fibrotic tissue from main trunk to subsegmental arteries. It is important to inspect and free all the pulmonary vascular segments: it has been demonstrated that hemodynamic improvement and prognosis are proportional to number of reopened segments [16, 17].

On the other side, good surgical results could be burdened by extensive parenchymal edema due to a large re-perfused territory. Reperfusion edema occurs in up to 20% of cases and, probably, it is the most common complication after PEA. The pathogenesis is not completely explained but it is due to a dysfunction of capillary-alveolar membrane at the level of previously occluded territories. Different degrees of reperfusion edema can be managed with a stepwise approach: in uncomplicated initial stages, optimization of mechanical ventilatory support and maximization of diuretic therapy should be adequate. However, in complicated cases, with massive lung involvement and refractory respiratory failure, bridge-to-recovery ECLS is often necessary [10, 14].

Another technical challenge of PEA is to carry out the endarterectomy not too deep, avoiding transmural lesions that can cause parenchymal bleeding: it is a rare, but life-threatening complication, with a prevalence between 0.5 and 2% of cases. Technical problems, the fragility of the endarterectomies wall and the presence of parenchymal infarcted areas may contribute to hemorrhagic complications after reperfusion [18, 19]. Precautionary measures include a careful endarterectomy and proper pulmonary venting during reperfusion/rewarming period. Moreover, an intraoperative double check is routinely performed, first with the "bubble technique" during gentle ventilation and then with bronchoscopy during re-warming, once a normal core temperature is reached. Typically, bleeding starts just after weaning from CPB, because of the increase in pulmonary pressure. If bleeding is mild, complete re-coagulation could be sufficient. In case of severe parenchymal or endobronchial hemorrhage, ECLS with bridge-to-recovery strategy represents a life-saving tool, associated with mechanical and/or pharmacological local hemostasis and optimal reversal of post-CPB coagulopathy [19, 20].

Residual PH after PEA ranges from 8.2% to 44.5% [21]. It is due to micro-vasculopathy, incomplete revascularization of pulmonary vascular tree or both; predictors of residual PH have been reported: high preoperative PVR, distal surgical material, and associated medical conditions (splenectomy, ventriculoatrial shunt, permanent central intravenous lines, inflammatory bowel disease, and osteomyelitis). Unsuccessful procedures with persistent PH in addition to surgical trauma (long CPB time, DHCA, reperfusion lung injury) can lead to an RV overload and failure requiring ECLS [10, 22, 23].

In summary, clinical indications for ECLS can be divided into different groups:

- those with proximal occlusion and good surgical results that suffer massive parenchymal edema due to a large reperfused territory;

- those with a bad preoperative hemodynamic profile, RV failure and distal occlusion, who have a minimal decrease of PH after satisfactory PEA. In these cases, the small and peripheral disease is the main cause of failure;

- those with parenchymal bleeding secondary to technical problems and fragility of the denuded vessels, and the presence of areas of infarcted lung parenchyma which may contribute to hemorrhage after reperfusion.

3. Surgical strategies and ECLS setup

Many centers reported their experience in PEA, focusing on perioperative ECLS: there is no consensus on the best strategy, because of multiple possible indications and approaches, but many authors recommend a prompt, aggressive treatment with ECLS before severe end-stage organ hypoperfusion, possibly with a tailored approach [15, 18].

Table 1 summarizes the most relevant series in the last two decades.

ECLS can be set up as veno-venous (VV) or veno-arterial (VA) support. Isolated potentially reversible respiratory failure requiring VV-ECLS is an infrequent scenario, because of the aforementioned vitious circles triggered by complications after PEA: often respiratory failure (hypoxia), high PVR and increased lung stiffness offers an excessive hemodynamic barrage to RV, leading to heart failure.

The group of San Diego advocates the use of VV-ECLS in selected patients because of its technical advantages (physiologic flow and no influence on ventricular pre- and after-load, simple and quick implantation; peripheral and percutaneous access, avoiding redo-sternotomy; on the other side, it is burdened by a significant risk of bleeding, infectious and thromboembolic complications if support is

References	Year	Study design	No. of cases (%)	Strategy		Timing
Thistlethwaite PA et al. [14]	2006	Retrospective	20/1790 (1.1)	VV	Peripheral	Post
Ogino O et al. [18]	2006	Retrospective	8/88 (9.1)	VA	Peripheral	Post
Berman M et al. [24]	2008	Retrospective	7/127 (5.5)	VA	Central	Post
Nierlich P et al. [9]	2015	Retrospective	31/161 (19.3)	VA	Peripheral	Pre-Post
Boulate et al. [11]	2016	Retrospective	31/829 (3.7)	VA-VV	Central-Peripheral	Post
Donahoe L et al. [15]	2016	Retrospective	6/144 (4.0)	VA-VV	Central-Peripheral	Post
Guth S et al. [19]	2016	Retrospective	16/396 (4.0) 8/396 (2.0)	VA	Central	Post
Kelava M et al. [12]	2018	Retrospective	14/150 (9.3)	VA-VV		Pre-Post
Martin-Suarez S et al. [10]	2019	Retrospective	19/154 (12.3)	VA-VV	Central-Peripheral	Post
Sugiyama K et al. [25]	2019	Retrospective	4/35 (11)	VA		Post

VA veno-arterial, VV veno-venous.

Table 1.
Literature reports on type of strategy.

prolonged) [14]. Standard VV-ECLS is achieved through bi-femoral or jugulo-femoral cannulation; the use of dual lumen cannula (Avalon Elite, Avalon Laboratories, Rancho Dominguez, CA, USA) reduces invasiveness and further simplifies the procedure.

Particular care must be taken in titrating pump flow in order to increase oxygen delivery without any recirculation between the drainage and reinfusion cannulas.

VA-ECLS is preferred by many centers because it provides efficient RV unloading, and reduces transpulmonary flow, parenchymal edema, and/or bleeding. Furthermore, the increased afterload due to arterial inflow improves the filling and diastolic performance of the left ventricle, as well as preventing RV distension and leftward septal shift. But there are some drawbacks, especially in case of peripheral setting, such as unphysiological retrograde perfusion that is at high risk of stroke, "Harlequin syndrome" and limb ischemia [9–11, 24].

Cannulation could be peripheral or central. The standard peripheral setting involves femoro-femoral cannulation, but other cannulation sites such as the subclavian artery can be a viable option: an upper extremity configuration allows mobility and even re-habilitation, especially in case of BTT strategy. Technically, femoro-femoral approach is a straightforward procedure that can be easily done in stable conditions while CPB is already ongoing. If feasible, the chest can be definitively closed, reducing the risk of infection and supporting recovery in more physiological conditions. Moreover, cannulas can be removed in the ICU. Of course, troubles with lower limb ischemia or other vascular complications may occur and periodically checked and eventually treated with distal reperfusion [9, 10].

Furthermore, considering flows ranging from 2.5–4 L/min, external oxygenator allows reduction of the mechanical ventilation protecting impaired alveolo-capillary units from barotrauma or high oxygen exposure.

If ECLS is started in the operating room for impossible weaning from CPB, some authors suggest central VA configuration, because it decreases RV afterload, and ensures a pulsatile blood flow into the lung vessels, avoiding overflow episodes during the early postoperative period. Preventive VA-ECMO should be a reasonable BTR strategy that mitigates the negative effects of both critical pulmonary reperfusion syndrome and severe RVF, after PEA procedures [11, 15].

In summary, VV-ECLS should be the treatment of choice for pulmonary reperfusion injury, manifested as pulmonary edema with preserved right heart function, particularly if it occurs in the intensive care unit after PEA. For persistent residual PH and ongoing RV failure, central VA ECLS was excellent providing both oxygenation and effective unloading of the right heart and pulmonary vessels [15].

Regardless of the management strategy, unfortunately, ECLS is burdened by bleeding, infective, and thromboembolic complications, thus patients must be weaned from ECLS as soon as possible.

4. Results and outcomes

The need for postoperative ECLS ranges between 1 and 19%; incidence tends to decrease with experience and in high-volume centers. Mean support time ranges between 4 and 5 days. Successful weaning rate range between 43 and 100% [10, 11, 14, 15, 18, 19, 24, 25].

The main risk factor for ECLS was high PVR often associated with distal thromboembolic disease (Jamieson type 4), while predictors of mortality after ECLS were elder age, high PVR, RV failure, reperfusion injuries, and parenchymal bleeding [9–11, 14, 15].

Considering postoperative hemodynamics, PVR was significantly better in non-ECLS patients [9, 24, 25].

Only two studies reported postoperative BTT strategy: in these cases, survival was about 50% and, according to Boulate and colleagues, survival was similar in BTT and BTR strategies [9, 11].

In general, in comparison with patients not requiring ECLS, long-term survival was significantly lower in ECLS patients [9].

On the other side, early hemodynamic improvement in patients with successful BTR-ECLS persisted in the midterm, confirming the benefit of PEA also in patients with severe CTEPH. This observation is consistent with microvascular disease reversal within a few weeks after PEA as previously suggested in human and animal models [11].

Interestingly, in case of parenchymal bleeding Guth and colleagues tailored the approach to reaching excellent results with 100% of successful weaning: prompt institution of ECLS systems with heparin-coated circuits instead of conventional extracorporeal circulatory support during PEA surgery allows complete restoration of blood coagulation with protamine with a minimal risk of clot formation inside the oxygenator: the majority of patients were treated in the operating theater with very short term support and avoiding long-term complications.

In our experience, ECLS was needed in 12.3% of patients who underwent PEA. The duration of ECMO was 11 ± 8 days and successful weaning was achieved in 52.6%

of cases, of these 70% were discharged. Also, in our experience, high PVR was associated with a high risk of ECLS. Surprisingly, the PAPs were lower in the nonsurvivor group: this could be a flag of RV dysfunction function, not able to produce adequate pulmonary flow and pulsatility [10].

5. Conclusions

In conclusion, ECLS represents a successful treatment option for patients who experience cardiopulmonary failure after PEA: patients with a more compromised preoperative hemodynamic profile and distal thromboembolic lesions are at high risk of the need for ECLS. Multiple strategies are available for treatment and there is no consensus about the optimal approach: timely and tailored approaches offer the best results.

Author details

Antonio Loforte[1*], Gregorio Gliozzi[1], Giulio Giovanni Cavalli[1], Carlo Mariani[1], Luca Botta[1], Nazzareno Galiè[2], Davide Pacini[1] and Sofia Martin-Suarez[1]

1 Cardiac Surgery Department, S. Orsola University Hospital, IRCCS Bologna, Alma Mater Studiorum University of Bologna, Bologna, Italy

2 Cardiology Department, S. Orsola University Hospital, IRCCS Bologna, Alma Mater Studiorum University of Bologna, Bologna, Italy

*Address all correspondence to: antonioloforte@yahoo.it

References

[1] Ende-Verhaar YM, Cannegieter SC, Noordegraaf AV, Delcroix M, Pruszczyk P, Mairuhu ATA, et al. Incidence of chronic thromboembolic pulmonary hypertension after acute pulmonary embolism: A contemporary view of the published literature. European Respiratory Journal. 2017;**49**:1601792. DOI: 10.1183/13993003.01792-2016

[2] Simonneau G, Gatzoulis MA, Adatia I, Celermajer D, Denton C, Ghofrani A, et al. Updated clinical classification of pulmonary hypertension. Journal of the American College of Cardiology. 2013;**62**:D34-D41. DOI: 10.1016/j.jacc.2013.10.029

[3] Pepke-Zaba J, Ghofrani HA, Hoeper MM. Medical management of chronic thromboembolic pulmonary hypertension. European Respiratory Review. 2017;**26**:160107. DOI: 10.1183/16000617.0107-2016

[4] Simonneau G, Torbicki A, Dorfmüller P, Kim N. The pathophysiology of chronic thromboembolic pulmonary hypertension. European Respiratory Review. 2017;**26**:160112. DOI: 10.1183/16000617.0112-2016

[5] Simonneau G, Dorfmüller P, Guignabert C, Mercier O, Humbert M. Chronic thromboembolic pulmonary hypertension: The magic of pathophysiology. Annals of Cardiothoracic Surgery. 2022;**11**:106-119. DOI: 10.21037/acs-2021-pte-10

[6] Martin-Suarez S, Loforte A, Cavalli GG, Gliozzi G, Botta L, Mariani C, et al. Therapeutic alternatives in chronic thromboembolic pulmonary hypertension: From pulmonary endarterectomy to balloon pulmonary angioplasty to medical therapy. State of the art from a multidisciplinary team. Annals of Cardiothoracic Surgery. 2022;**11**:120-127. DOI: 10.21037/acs-2021-pte-23

[7] Delcroix M, Torbicki A, Gopalan D, Sitbon O, Klok FA, Lang I, et al. ERS statement on chronic thromboembolic pulmonary hypertension. European Respiratory Journal. 2021;**57**:2002828. DOI: 10.1183/13993003.02828-2020

[8] Jenkins D, Madani M, Fadel E, D'Armini AM, Mayer E. Pulmonary endarterectomy in the management of chronic thromboembolic pulmonary hypertension. European Respiratory Review. 2017;**26**:160111. DOI: 10.1183/16000617.0111-2016

[9] Nierlich P, Ristl R. Perioperative extracorporeal membrane oxygenation bridging in patients undergoing pulmonary endarterectomy. Interactive Cardiovascular and Thoracic Surgery. 2016;**22**:181-187. DOI: 10.1093/icvts/ivv318

[10] Martin-Suarez S, Gliozzi G, Fiorentino M, Loforte A, Ghigi V, di Camillo M, et al. Role and management of extracorporeal life support after surgery of chronic thromboembolic pulmonary hypertension. Annals of Cardiothoracic Surgery. 2019;**8**:84-92. DOI: 10.21037/acs.2019.01.02

[11] Boulate D, Mercier O, Mussot S, Fabre D, Stephan F, Haddad F, et al. Extracorporeal life support after pulmonary endarterectomy as a bridge to recovery or transplantation: Lessons from 31 consecutive patients. Annals of Thoracic Surgery. 2016;**102**:P260-P268. DOI: 10.1016/j.athoracsur.2016.01.103

[12] Kelava M, Koprivanac M, Smedira N, Mihaljevic T, Alfirevic A. Extracorporeal membrane oxygenation in pulmonary endarterectomy patients. Journal of Cardiothoracic and Vascular Anesthesia. 2019;**33**:60-69. DOI: 10.1053/j.jvca.2018.06.025

[13] D'Armini AM, Morsolini M, Mattiucci G, Grazioli V, Pin M, Valentini A, et al. Pulmonary endarterectomy for distal chronic thromboembolic pulmonary hypertension. Journal of Thoracic and Cardiovascular Surgery. 2014;**148**:1005-1011. DOI: 10.1016/j.jtcvs.2014.06.052

[14] Thistlethwaite PA, Madani MM, Kemp AD, Hartley M, Auger WR, Jamieson SW. Venovenous extracorporeal life support after pulmonary endarterectomy: Indications, techniques, and outcomes. Annals of Thoracic Surgery. 2006;**82**:2139-2145. DOI: 10.1016/j.athoracsur.2006.07.020

[15] Donahoe L, Granton J, McRae K, Thenganatt J, Moric J, Keshavjee S, et al. Role of extracorporeal life support after pulmonary endarterectomy: A single-Centre experience. Interactive Cardiovascular and Thoracic Surgery. 2016;**23**:74-78. DOI: 10.1093/icvts/ivw075

[16] Pin M, Vanini B, Sciortino A, Grazioli V, Merli V, Celentano A, et al. Pulmonary endarterectomy: Relationship between Total reopened branches and outcomes. The Journal of Heart and Lung Transplantation. 2018;**37**:S26. DOI: 10.1016/j.healun.2018.01.043

[17] Jamieson SW, Kapelanski DP. Pulmonary endarterectomy. Current Problems in Surgery. 2000;**37**:167-252. DOI: 10.1016/s0011-3840(00)80005-2

[18] Ogino H, Ando M, Matsuda H, Minatoya K, Sasaki H, Nakanishi N, et al. Japanese single-center experience of surgery for chronic thromboembolic pulmonary hypertension. Annals of Thoracic Surgery. 2006;**82**:P630-P636. DOI: 10.1016/j.athoracsur.2006.03.121

[19] Guth S, Wiedenroth CB, Wollenschläger M, Richter MJ, Ghofrani HA, Arlt M, et al. Short-term venoarterial extracorporeal membrane oxygenation for massive endobronchial hemorrhage after pulmonary endarterectomy. Journal of Thoracic and Cardiovascular Surgery. 2018;**155**:P643-P649. DOI: 10.1016/j.jtcvs.2017.09.045

[20] Morsolini M, Azzaretti A, Orlandoni G, D'Armini AM. Airway bleeding during pulmonary endarterectomy: The "bubbles" technique. Journal of Thoracic and Cardiovascular Surgery. 2013;**145**:P1409-P1410. DOI: 10.1016/j.jtcvs.2012.12.045

[21] Brookes JDL, Li C, Chung STW, Brookes EM, Williams ML, McNamara N, et al. Pulmonary thromboendarterectomy for chronic thromboembolic pulmonary hypertension: A systematic review. Annals of Cardiothoracic Surgery. 2022;**11**:68-81. DOI: 10.21037/acs-2021-pte-25

[22] Godinas L, Verbelen T, Delcroix M. Residual pulmonary hypertension after pulmonary thromboendarterectomy: Incidence, pathogenesis and therapeutic options. Annals of Cardiothoracic Surgery. 2022;**11**:163-165. DOI: 10.21037/acs-2021-pte-11

[23] Loforte A, Comentale G, Gliozzi G, Cavalli GG, Pacini D, Martin-Suarez S. Mechanical circulatory supports after pulmonary thrombo-endarterectomy: Why, when and how. Annals of Cardiothoracic Surgery. 2022;**11**:169-171. DOI: 10.21037/acs-2021-pte-16

[24] Berman M, Tsui S, Vuylsteke A, Snell A, Colah S, Latimer R, et al. Successful extracorporeal membrane oxygenation support after pulmonary Thromboendarterectomy. Annals of Thoracic Surgery. 2008;**86**:P1261-P1267. DOI: 10.1016/j.athoracsur.2008.06.037

[25] Sugiyama K, Suzuki S, Fujiyoshi T, Koizumi N, Sato M, Ogino H. Extracorporeal membrane oxygenation after pulmonary endarterectomy for chronic thromboembolic pulmonary hypertension. Journal of Cardiac Surgery. 2019;**34**:428-434. DOI: 10.1111/jocs.14052

Chapter 6

Left Ventricular Unloading in v-a ECLS Patients

Gaik Nersesian, Daniel Lewin, Pia Lanmüller, Sascha Ott and Evgenij Potapov

Abstract

The v-a ECLS is an effective approach for mechanical circulatory support, however, it is associated with several disadvantages. An increased afterload generated by a pump outflow leads to a left ventricular (LV) distension, pulmonary congestion, and lung edema on one hand and impairs myocardial perfusion on the other. In this chapter, we will discuss the rationality as well as different techniques for LV unloading during v-a ECLS support.

Keywords: ECLS, LV unloading, ECMELLA, Impella, IABP, venting

1. Introduction

V-a ECLS represents an effective rescue therapy in patients suffering circulatory failure. The mechanical circulatory support (MCS) with a v-a ECLS can be rapidly established, achieving a blood flow of up to 9.9 L/min and simultaneous blood oxygenation and decarboxylation [1]. Uncomplicated placement, reasonable costs, and the possibility to implant a v-a ECLS during an ongoing cardiopulmonary resuscitation (eCPR) have made it a widely used mobile tool for first-line MCS [2].

Despite these alluring benefits v-a ECLS is an invasive approach and has its side effects, which have to be taken into consideration [2]. One of the significant disadvantages of the system is an increased afterload of the LV generated by the pump outflow [3]. In patients with severely impaired cardiac function, this can cause LV distention and ballooning, increasing the myocardial oxygen consumption, and impairing the coronary perfusion at the same time [2]. In addition, increased left heart end-diastolic pressure leads to pulmonary congestion and edema, with the consequence of respiratory failure [3]. All these factors limit the potential benefits of the v-a ECLS and complicate circulatory weaning [3]. Temporary MCS with v-a ECLS can impair ventricular recovery regardless of the severity of myocardial damage [4].

In order to prevent an LV distention on v-a ECLS, several approaches can be established: LV unloading via passive LV venting, creation of an ASD, or with a microaxial catheter-based Impella pump. Alternatively, LV afterload can be decreased by using a combination of ECLS with an intra-aortic balloon counterpulsation (IABP).

2. Passive venting

LV venting can be achieved through the placement of an additional inflow cannula draining the left atrium or LV into the venous side of the ECLS. In the case of post-cardiotomy patients, the venting cannula is usually placed in the left ventricle via the right superior pulmonary vein and then connected by a Y-tubing to the venous drainage line of the ECLS circuit [5]. Alternatively, the venting cannula may be directly placed into LV via the left ventricular apex, with a subsequent subxiphoid tunneling and externalization [5]. Another possibility is the direct placement of the cannula into the pulmonary artery [3].

In rare cases, an iatrogenic atrial septal defect (ASD) can be created in order to achieve passive drainage of the left atrium (LA) via a venous cannula placed in the right atrium [6]. This approach can be performed both surgically or by a percutaneous blade and balloon atrioseptostomy and is considered more as rescue therapy rather than a standard approach [6].

3. Percutaneous venting

Alternatively, in patients with a closed chest on peripheral v-a ECLS left ventricular apical cannulation can be performed through a left anterolateral thoracotomy. This approach requires high surgical expertise due to potential LV damage, coronary injury, and a high risk of bleeding [5].

Furthermore, percutaneous approaches for LV unloading are available [5]. The TandemHeart system (LivaNova PLC, London, UK) uses a single-stage cannula, which can be placed percutaneously in the LA through an atrial septal puncture providing LV unloading on mechanical circulatory support [7].

The specially designed Bio-Medicus NextGen two-stage cannula (Medtronic PLC., Dublin, Ireland) can be applied in order to obtain both left-sided venting and venous drainage simultaneously. For this approach, the cannula is placed via a femoral vein with its tip advanced into the LA; the venous drainage is achieved by a second inflow positioned in the inferior vena cava [7]. The cannulation in both cases is performed in a catheterization lab or hybrid operation room under fluoroscopic and/or echocardiographic guidance. The major drawback of this method is ASD remains after decannulation. In the vast majority of cases, the iatrogenic ASD has no hemodynamic influence, however, can become relevant in patients undergoing a LVAD implantation [7].

4. LV unloading during v-a ECLS employing IABP

A combination of v-a ECLS with an intra-aortic balloon pump (IABP) can be applied for LV unloading. The use of IABP can decrease LV afterload during systole, increase diastolic blood pressure and coronary blood flow, and significantly improve survival in ECLS patients [5, 8]. However, since the publication of the IABP-SHOCK II Trial, where no survival benefit for IABP application in cardiogenic shock patients could be demonstrated, the use of IABP is decreasing [9]. The effect of the IABP on LV unloading depends on a degree of LV contractility—the less contractility, the less unloading [3]. Therefore, in patients for whom LV requires maximal unloading, the IABP does not work [9]. Nevertheless, IABP remains a feasible option for patients with mechanical aortic valves, since Impella unloading is technically not possible, and passive LV unloading may preclude LV ejection and, therefore, carry a high risk for mechanical aortic valve thrombosis [10]. Further, in patients with mobile LV thrombus precluding Impella unloading, IABP remains a feasible alternative [10, 11].

5. ECMELLA approach

Implantation of microaxial catheter-based devices, such as Impella (Abiomed Inc., Danvers, MA, and USA), provides temporary MCS with simultaneous LV

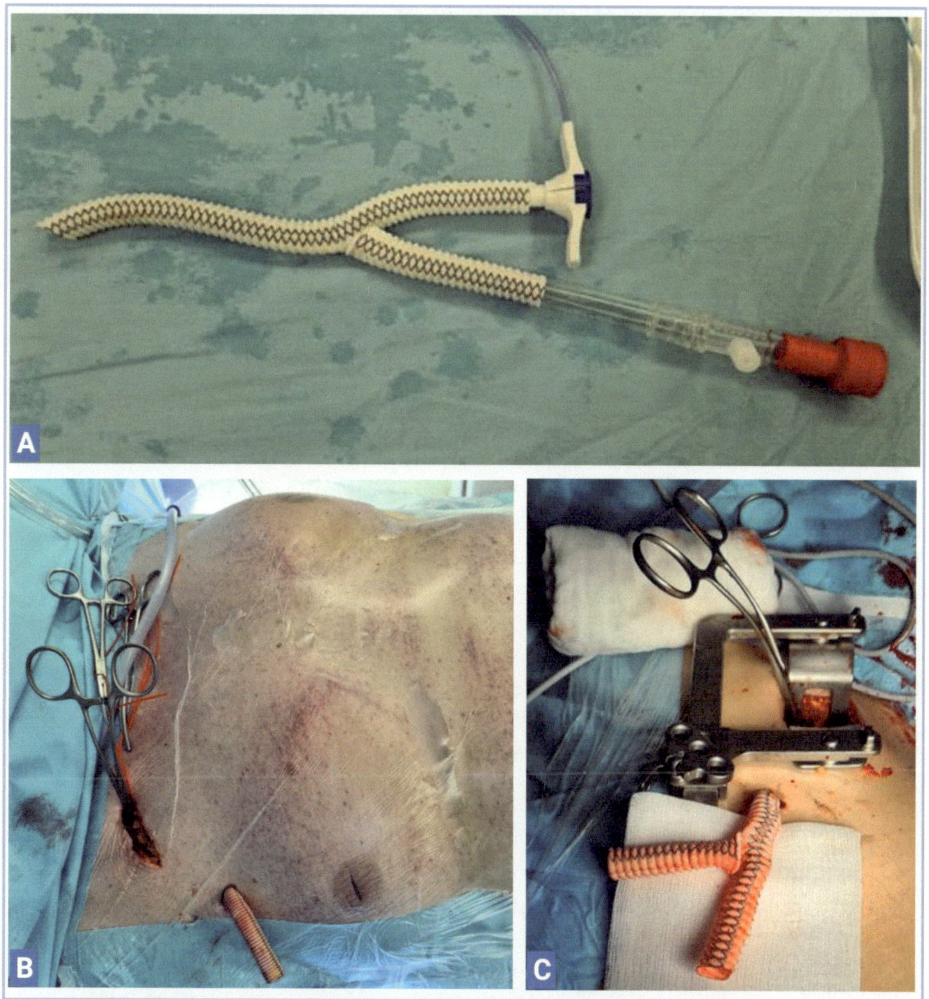

A. 10 mm Y-shaped vascular graft prosthesis with an Impella 5.0/5.5 introducer and arterial cannula of the v-a ECLS
B. Simple vascular graft prosthesis anastomosed to the right axillary artery used for a surgical Impella implantation
C. Y-shaped graft anastomosed to the right axillary artery as a part of ECMELLA 2.0/2.1 approach

Figure 1.
Single arterial access ECMELLA cannulation.

unloading [12]. The combination of Impella and v-a ECLS, so-called ECMELLA approach provides advanced cardiopulmonary support in cardiogenic shock patients and has been demonstrated to significantly improve the outcomes compared to ECLS use alone [4, 11, 12]. Impella devices (Impella 2.5, CP, 5.0, and 5.5) are directly placed in the LV via the aortic valve, providing an anterograde blood flow and unloading in contrast to an ECLS [1, 2, 12]. Thereby, Impella within the ECMELLA approach enhances the support concept to a cardiocirculatory, rather than just a circulatory support system [13].

The Impella 2.5 and CP devices are placed percutaneously and support the hemodynamic with 2.5 up to 4.3 L/min. The surgically implanted Impella 5.0 and 5.5 models are able to generate full circulatory support with up to 5.5 L/min of blood flow. In the case of ECMELLA approach, an Impella flow of 1–2 L/min is usually enough for a sufficient LV unloading [10]. However, the application of more powerful Impella models can be beneficial, since it allows a de-escalation therapy meaning gradual ECLS weaning and explantation during increased Impella support and patients' mobilization [14].

Nevertheless, ECMELLA is associated with some vascular complications [4]. The necessity of additional arterial access increases the risk of access site bleeding, hematoma, dissections, and infections [4]. The ECMELLA 2.0 technique aims to reduce that issues, by utilization of a single arterial access technique. In this case, a Y-shaped vascular prosthesis is anastomosed to the patient's subclavian artery. One branch of the graft is used for Impella insertion, while the arterial cannula of ECLS is placed via the second side branch (**Figure 1**) [13, 15]. This method allows advanced cardiopulmonary support with flow rates above 10 L/min, providing biventricular unloading at the same time [13]. Another major advantage of this technique is the possibility for bedside de-escalation and ECLS explanation, which can be performed in local anesthesia and does not require surgical re-opening of the wound [10, 16].

Further improvement of the single-site ECMELLA approach is the ECMELLA 2.1 technique, with the percutaneous cannulation of the jugular vein for blood drainage. This approach allows patients' mobilization on ongoing support for an extended period of time (**Table 1**) [17].

Parameter	Passive vent	Percutaneous vent	ECLS + IABP	ECMELLA
Access	Sternotomy/ thoracotomy	Percutaneous	Percutaneous	Percutaneous/ surgical cut-down
Additional hemodynamic support	N/A	N/A	N/A	2.5–5.5 L/min
Size	12–18 Fr	15–21 Fr*	7.5 Fr	12–24 Fr
Costs	*	**	**	***
Mobilization	No	No	Possible (axillary cannulation)	Yes for ECMELLA 2.0/2.1
Explantation	Surgical	Surgical/ Percutaneous	Percutaneous	Surgical/ Percutaneous

**For Bio-Medicus NextGen cannulas.*

Table 1.
Comparison of different LV unloading strategies.

6. Discussion

6.1 Timing of unloading

Various studies have demonstrated the advantages of LV unloading in ECLS patients. However, the timing and patient selection still represent a point of high debate among advanced heart failure specialists [4, 10]. The propensity score matched the multicenter study from Schrage et al., which demonstrated that LV unloading (with Impella) initiated before or shortly after the v-a ECMO implantation significantly improves survival compared to v-a ECLS alone [4]. However, a subgroup analysis of those patients who underwent delayed unloading (>2 h since ECLS), revealed no significant survival benefits [4]. Still, there is a point of discussion if the LV unloading has to be performed simultaneously in ECLS or if a delayed approach is more optimal in a clinical setting. The propensity score matched the study from Grandin et al., which demonstrated that patients who undergo an upright LV unloading have no differences in regard to on-support or in-hospital mortality but a lower incidence of renal injury compared to the delayed unloading cohort [11]. Moreover, initiation of a LV unloading after a period of v-a ECLS exposure might be associated with increased procedural risk and technical difficulties with the placement of an additional device [4, 11].

6.2 System choice

Another important point of the LV unloading strategy is the choice of the system. Several important aspects should be taken into consideration during the decision-making process:

- Approximate duration of MCS, potential weaning
- Vascular access possibilities
- Complication profile
- Availability of each system and costs

The current evidence-based data have demonstrated that the LV unloading in v-a ECLS patients improve the patients' outcomes [1, 4, 11, 12, 18]. However, no general recommendation or guideline on the technique of LV unloading exists [3]. The decision-making is often based on the expertise of the performing surgeon or interventional cardiologist and the internal standardized operational protocols of each clinic [3].

Although the LV unloading via an additional inflow cannula placed through the apex of the right superior pulmonary vein represents the most cost-effective and simplified approach, it is predominantly reserved for patients with central ECLS [3]. Since it requires a sternotomy or thoracotomy, it might be associated with an increased risk for collateral surgical damage [3]. Another major disadvantage is the necessity for surgical removal of the cannula for weaning. In this constellation, the utilization of specialized percutaneous venting cannulas represents a preferable and flexible solution and has been increasingly applied in recent years [7].

Currently, the vast majority of patients receive LV unloading with either IABP or Impella devices [11]. Both approaches provide similar survival benefits, however, have different complications and hemodynamic profiles [11]. The implantation site bleeding and vascular injury remain the major disadvantage for LV unloading since the addition of extra arterial access increases the risk for complications [4, 11]. However, in the case of an IABP it is significantly lower due to the size of the used catheter (7.5 Fr compared to 14 Fr in Impella CP in devices) [3]. Finally, yet importantly, the ECMELLA therapy is associated with significantly higher costs compared to LV unloading with a venting cannula or an IABP [3].

Despite its invasiveness, the ECMELLA approach has some unique advantages which have to be taken into consideration during the decision-making process [13]. The ECMELLA provides the highest level of temporary cardiopulmonary support currently available in surgical armaments [15, 19]. In patients suffering from systemic inflammation response syndrome and consecutive vasoplegia as a sequel of, or coincidently with, severe cardiogenic shock or after CPR, optimal flow rates of up to 11 L/min or even more might be necessary [15, 20, 21]. ECMELLA allows a controlled stepwise support reduction and de-escalation strategy: v-a ECLS explantation with further Impella support, which achieves a reduction of ECLS-related complications in patients requiring prolonged support [1]. The recently developed single arterial access ECMELLA 2.1 includes advantages of high flow support, patients' mobilization, and bedside explantation, with no need for a renewed exploration of the implantation site [13, 15, 17].

6.3 Perspectives

Currently, two randomized controlled trials investigating the impact of LV unloading in v-a ECLS patients have been launched: the REVERSE (NCT03431467) trial from the University of Pennsylvania and ANCHOR (NCT04184635) trial guided by the Hôpital Pitié Salpétrière from Paris. The REVERSE trial aims to investigate the impact of Impella CP as a vent in v-a ECLS patients, while the unloading has to be initiated within 10 h after implantation of the v-a ECLS. Planning to recruit 96 patients, the first results are expected in 2025. The ANCHOR trial compares 200 patients with acute myocardial infarction-related CS (AMICS) treated with v-a ECLS + IABP vs. a control group without tMCS. The finishing is scheduled for the end of 2024. However, no prospective study investigating different LV unloading strategies is currently available.

The self-expandable catheter-based microaxial pumps represent a promising improvement in MCS [22]. This technology allows percutaneous insertion of narrow-profiled devices, which expand during support aiming to reduce the risk for vascular complications and hemolysis by minimizing the shear stress on blood cells [22]. The HeartMate Percutaneous Heart Pump (PHP, Abbott Vascular, Santa Clara, CA, and US) was the first pump that was deployed via a 14 Fr femoral arterial sheath and delivered a self-expanding 24 Fr nitinol cannula and impeller across the aortic valve [22]. However, due to a high incidence of device malfunctions, the HartMate PHP was not implemented in clinical practice [22]. The recently presented Impella ECP (Abiomed Inc., Danvers, MA, and US) device has a 9 Fr catheter and an up to 18 Fr size expandable body. Currently, the ECP trial (NCT05334784) investigating the effect of the device on patients with high-risk coronary interventions is scheduled. Both devices were originally designed for periprocedural support during high-risk interventions (max. 6–12 h); however, self-expandable Impeller pumps can be potentially used for prolonged support in cardiogenic shock patients in future (**Table 2**) [22].

Study, first author	Year	Investigated cohorts	Outcomes
Retrospective studies			
Gass et al. [8]	2014	135 v-a ECLS + IABP	Overall, in-hospital survival of 57.8%, high incidence of access site bleeding.
Pappalardo et al. [12]	2017	42 v-a ECLS vs. 21 ECMELLA*	Significantly better survival for ECMELLA, no difference in bleeding complications.
Schrage et al. [4]	2020	255 v-a ECLS vs. 255 ECMELLA*	Significantly better survival for ECMELLA, more access-related bleeding, hemolysis, and need for renal replacement therapy in ECMELLA group.
Tongers et al. [19]	2020	69 ECMELLA	Early MCS escalation (ECMELLA) rapidly stabilized patients, reducing number and doses of catecholamines, and improves hemodynamics.
Grandin et al. [11]	2022	3399 ECLS patients with LV unloading vs. 9335 without	Significantly decreased in-hospital mortality for LV unloading group at the expense of more complications, including hemolysis and cannulation site bleeding.
Prospective randomized trials			
REVERSE Trial	2018–2025	96 v-a ECLS with Impella CP as vent	Patients randomized to the experimental arm will have an Impella CP implanted in addition to v-a ECLS <10 h since the institution of v-a ECLS
ANCHOR Trial	2019–2024	200 patients v-a ECLS with IABP vs. 200 without tMCS	Experimental arm v-a ECLS + IABP instituted percutaneously as soon as possible. Control arm: Standard management of CS due to myocardial infarction, according to the current ESC guidelines. It is not recommended to use IABP support and no other tMCS devices are allowed.

**Cohorts after propensity score matching.*

Table 2.
Important studies on LV unloading in v-a ECLS patients.

7. Conclusion

Active LV unloading in v-a ECLS patients improves survival, however, the costs of more vascular complications, bleeding, and hemolysis. Prospective randomized trials comparing different LV unloading approaches are required in order to optimize the treatment. Perspective devices and equipment might reduce the complications associated with LV unloading and ease clinical management.

Author details

Gaik Nersesian[1,2*], Daniel Lewin[1], Pia Lanmüller[1,2], Sascha Ott[3,4] and Evgenij Potapov[1,2]

1 Department of Cardiothoracic and Vascular Surgery, German Heart Center Berlin, Berlin, Germany

2 DZHK (German Centre for Cardiovascular Research), Berlin, Germany

3 Department of Cardiac Anesthesiology and Intensive Care Medicine, German Heart Center Berlin, Berlin, Germany

4 Department of Cardiac Anesthesiology and Intensive Care Medicine, Charité-Universitätsmedizin Berlin, Berlin, Germany

*Address all correspondence to: nersesian@dhzb.de

References

[1] Tschope C, Van Linthout S, Klein O, et al. Mechanical unloading by fulminant myocarditis: LV-IMPELLA, ECMELLA, BI-PELLA, and PROPELLA concepts. Journal of Cardiovascular Translational Research. 2019;**12**:116-123

[2] Nersesian G, Hennig F, Muller M, et al. Temporary mechanical circulatory support for refractory heart failure: The German heart Center Berlin experience. Annals of Cardiothoracic Surgery. 2019;**8**:76-83

[3] Lusebrink E, Orban M, Kupka D, et al. Prevention and treatment of pulmonary congestion in patients undergoing venoarterial extracorporeal membrane oxygenation for cardiogenic shock. European Heart Journal. 2020;**41**:3753-3761

[4] Schrage B, Becher PM, Bernhardt A, et al. Left ventricular unloading is associated with lower mortality in patients with cardiogenic shock treated with Venoarterial extracorporeal membrane oxygenation: Results from an international. Multicenter Cohort Study. Circulation. 2020;**142**:2095-2106

[5] Brasseur A, Scolletta S, Lorusso R, Taccone FS. Hybrid extracorporeal membrane oxygenation. Journal of Thoracic Disease. 2018;**10**:S707-SS15

[6] Dahdouh Z, Roule V, Sabatier R, et al. Extra-corporeal life support, transradial thrombus aspiration and stenting, percutaneous blade and balloon atrioseptostomy, all as a bridge to heart transplantation to save one life. Cardiovascular Revascularization Medicine. 2012;**13**:241-245

[7] Orozco-Hernandez EJ, Ahmed MI, Von Meering G, et al. Femoral venoarterial extracorporeal membrane oxygenation using a novel biatrial cannula for venous drainage and left ventricular venting. Journal of Cardiac Surgery. 2020;**35**:3631-3633

[8] Gass A, Palaniswamy C, Aronow WS, et al. Peripheral venoarterial extracorporeal membrane oxygenation in combination with intra-aortic balloon counterpulsation in patients with cardiovascular compromise. Cardiology. 2014;**129**:137-143

[9] Thiele H, Zeymer U, Thelemann N, et al. Intraaortic balloon pump in cardiogenic shock complicating acute myocardial infarction: Long-term 6-year outcome of the randomized IABP-SHOCK II trial. Circulation. 2019;**139**:395-403

[10] Nersesian G, Potapov EV, Nelki V, et al. Propensity score-based analysis of 30-day survival in cardiogenic shock patients supported with different microaxial left ventricular assist devices. Journal of Cardiac Surgery. 2021;**36**:4141-4152

[11] Grandin EW, Nunez JI, Willar B, et al. Mechanical left ventricular unloading in patients undergoing Venoarterial extracorporeal membrane oxygenation. Journal of the American College of Cardiology. 2022;**79**:1239-1250

[12] Pappalardo F, Schulte C, Pieri M, et al. Concomitant implantation of Impella((R)) on top of veno-arterial extracorporeal membrane oxygenation may improve survival of patients with cardiogenic shock. European Journal of Heart Failure. 2017;**19**:404-412

[13] Montagner M, Nersesian G, Eulert-Grehn JJ, Wert L, Kempfert J,

Potapov E. Single arterial access ECMELLA: A new concept and step-by-step procedure. Multimedia Manual of Cardiothoracic Surgery. 2021:2021 [Online]

[14] Bertoldi LF, Pappalardo F, Lubos E, et al. Bridging INTERMACS 1 patients from VA-ECMO to LVAD via Impella 5.0: De-escalate and ambulate. Journal of Critical Care. 2020;**57**:259-263

[15] Eulert-Grehn JJ, Starck C, Kempfert J, Falk V, Potapov E. ECMELLA 2.0: Single arterial access technique for a staged approach in cardiogenic shock. The Annals of Thoracic Surgery. 2021;**111**:e135-e1e7

[16] Nersesian G, Tschope C, Spillmann F, et al. Prediction of survival of patients in cardiogenic shock treated by surgically implanted Impella 5+ short-term left ventricular assist device. Interactive Cardiovascular and Thoracic Surgery. 2020;**31**:475-482

[17] Bitargil M, Pham S, Haddad O, Sareyyupoglu B. Single arterial access for Ecpella and jugular venous cannulation provides full mobility on a status 1 heart transplant recipient. ESC Heart Failure. 2022;**9**:2003-2006

[18] Lorusso R, Meani P, Raffa GM, Kowalewski M. Extracorporeal membrane oxygenation and left ventricular unloading: What is the evidence? JTCVS Tech. 2022;**13**:101-114

[19] Tongers J, Sieweke JT, Kuhn C, et al. Early escalation of mechanical circulatory support stabilizes and potentially rescues patients in refractory cardiogenic shock. Circulation. Heart Failure. 2020;**13**:e005853

[20] Ott S, Lanmuller P, Nersesian G, et al. Management of increased systemic flow requirements in patients with left ventricular assist devices. Annals of Cardiothoracic Surgery. 2021;**10**:399-401

[21] Porizka M, Rulisek J, Flaksa M, et al. Dual veno-arterial extra-corporeal membrane oxygenation support in a patient with refractory hyperdynamic septic shock: A case report. Perfusion. 2022;**37**:306-310

[22] Kapur NK, Jorde UP, Sharma S, et al. Early experience with the HeartMate percutaneous heart pump from the SHIELD II trial. ASAIO Journal. 2022;**68**:492-497

Chapter 7

How to Do Weaning and Decannulation in Adult Cardiac

Pilje Kang

Abstract

If cardiac function is restored, we should consider discontinuing extracorporeal membrane oxygenation (ECMO) support. Except for patients who go to transplantation or ventricular assist device, the patient's condition should be evaluated steadily every day to determine and implement the weaning. Treatment interruption can be determined based on hemodynamic parameters, laboratory findings, and echocardiographic findings. Weaning is determined, and catheter removal is surgically removed or pressed by hand, and closure device is also used. Depending on the patient's condition and the decision of each center, the appropriate method can be selected. Since various complications may occur after removal, intensive observation should be carried out for a certain period of time.

Keywords: venous-arterial extracorporeal membrane oxygenation, weaning, weaning strategy, decannulation, ECMO

1. Introduction

Venous-arterial extracorporeal membrane oxygenation (VA ECMO) is applied in various situations [1]. Because ECMO is a process with some complications and side effects, it would be better to stop as soon as possible once the application target is achieved. If the patient's condition has not improved and the treatment is stopped, the patient's condition will deteriorate again. However, if ECMO support is maintained for too long, unnecessary complications caused by ECMO will occur, resulting in poor clinical results. Therefore, it is important to evaluate the patient well and stop applying ECMO when possible.

Weaning from VA-ECMO differs between centers and information about standardized weaning strategies are lacking. The weaning process still relies upon the single center's experience and individual clinical knowledge and skills.

The initial step in ECMO weaning is to identify the improvements in various aspects based on the recovery of cardiac function.

2. Weaning process

2.1 Factors of successful weaning

2.1.1 Hemodynamics parameters

The most easily obtained signal of when to start the ECMO weaning process is the patient's blood pressure. ECMO weaning can be considered if the patient's blood pressure and pulse pressure begin to increase even after applying the same ECMO flow and using the same inotropic medications. When the patient's blood pressure increases, the minimum mean arterial pressure is maintained at about 60 mmHg, and inotropes are gradually reduced or rarely used [2].

Substantial hemodynamic assessments may be needed during the weaning trial for critically ill patient monitoring. If the patient has a pulmonary arterial catheter, the pulmonary arterial catheter measurements provide key information regarding the right ventricle (RV) and left ventricle (LV) pre-loads [3]. To consider a patient for VA ECMO weaning, the hemodynamic variables with the pump off should be as follows: cardiac index >2.4 L/min/m2, mean blood pressure > 60 mmHg, pulmonary capillary wedge pressure < 18 mm Hg, and central venous pressure < 18 mmHg.

2.1.2 Laboratory findings

When considering ECMO weaning, laboratory findings should also be referred to, including blood tests for B-type natriuretic peptide, cardiac enzymes, lactate, liver function tests, and kidney function tests. A decreasing trend in these values rather than absolute values should be seen after ECMO support is withdrawn [4]. A few studies recommended that lactate and lactate clearance could aid for ECMO weaning [3].

2.1.3 Echocardiographic parameters

Echocardiography is a critical tool used to determine the recovery of both left ventricle and right ventricle function [5]. During ECMO support, performing echocardiography is recommended at least once a day as much as possible.

In several reports, ECMO weaning is likely when the following findings are observed [3, 4, 6, 7].

- Left ventricle ejection fraction (LV EF) ≥ 20 ~ 25%
- Aortic velocity-time integral (VTI) ≥ 10 ~ 12 cm
- Lateral mitral annulus peak systolic velocity (TDSa) ≥ 6 cm
- Small right ventricle (RV) dimensions, 3D RVEF ≥20 ~ 25%.

Both LV and RV size and function should be estimated during weaning of extracorporeal support and if distension and impending failure of either ventricle is noted, they may warrant termination of the weaning trial [6].

2.1.4 Other findings

In addition to myocardial recovery, end-organ recovery is essential. Pulmonary function should also not be compromised and pulmonary edema should be reduced as much as possible. A PaO2/FiO2 of ≥200, an oxygen fraction delivered by the extracorporeal circuit of 25%, and an oxygen fraction delivered by the ventilator circuit of 60% are rational for weaning trials. These measurements should be made with VA-ECMO blood flow at 1 ~ 1.5 L/min and a sweep gas flow rate of ≤1 L/min. Of note, if the patient

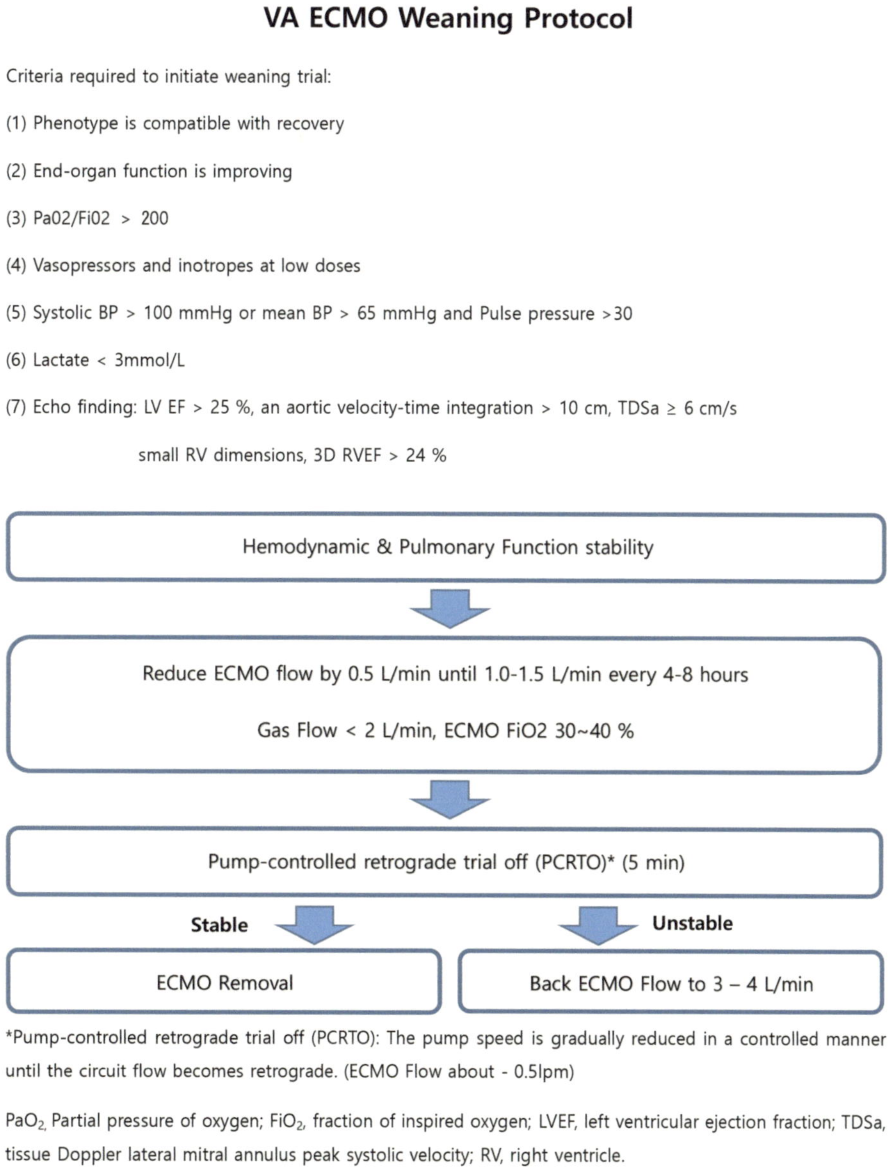

Figure 1.
VA ECMO weaning protocol.

experiences persistent pulmonary compromise but sufficient myocardial recovery could be achieved, switching to a veno-venous (VV)-ECMO should be considered [4].

If the findings listed above are observed, ECMO weaning is initiated.

2.2 Weaning trial

As mentioned earlier, there is no absolute way to determine the time for ECMO weaning. Each center or each person in charge has set and applied algorithms or protocols based on their own experience and knowledge. The patient should have estimated hemodynamic stability in the absence of or at low doses of vasoactive agents and pulsatile arterial waveform maintained for several hours. The ECMO flow is decreased to 60–70% of the initial flow rate for several minutes. It is then decreased to 30–40% for several minutes. Depending on the patient's condition, the ECMO weaning process may end within a day, or it may take several days. If the patient is stable in such a flow, it can be decreased to a minimum of 1–1.5 L/min and FiO2 in gas blender of <50–60% for several minutes. If no particular problem occurs during this process, ECMO removal can be considered. If mean blood pressure falls significantly and is continuously <50–60 mmHg during the trial, ECMO flow was returned to 100% of the initial flow and the trial is stopped. We propose the strategy we are using in our center in **Figure 1**.

2.2.1 The pump-controlled retrograde trial off (PCRTO)

Pump speed is steadily reduced in a controlled manner until circuit flow becomes retrograde, ensuring adequate RV filling and proper assessment of RV function. Since the circuit becomes an arteriovenous shunt, the revolving pump head acts as a resistor, preventing a significant drop in systemic vascular resistance during PCRTO. Patients can be considered ready for decannulation if the hemodynamic and echocardiographic criteria are met after a few minutes or hours [8]. Some researchers reported PCRTO to be a safe, simple, and reproducible approach for enabling a trial period while preserving the circuit during weaning from VA ECMO [9, 10]. In stable patients, PCRTO seems reasonable even if it is tested for 5–10 minutes without additional heparin or decannulation. However, in patients with low blood pressure or high vasoactive drugs with low ECMO flow, sufficient time spent on testing and removal will reduce the possibility of reinsertion.

3. Decannulation

Once the decision has been made to terminate ECMO, the cannulas are removed. Hemostasis can be achieved by extraction of the venous cannula from the femoral vein using a mattress suture and manual compression. Decannulation of arterial ECMO may be achieved by open surgical repair or *via* manual compression or using closing devices.

ECMO decannulation is related to the high risks of complications, such as bleeding, hematoma, pseudoaneurysm, thrombosis, and arterial-venous fistula. Bleeding complications occur after removal in 2%, with vascular complications generally up to 18% [11]. Frank Bidar et al. reported cannula-associated deep vein thrombosis occurred in 44 patients (41%), and arterial complications occurred in 15 (14%) (9 with acute leg ischemia, 1 with arteriovenous femoral fistula, and 5 with late femoral stenosis).

Vascular complications after ECMO decannulation can lead to prolong hospitalization and increase medical costs. Therefore, decannulation should be performed carefully and the patient's condition should be closely examined after cannula removal.

The selection of the cannula removal method is applied differently according to the condition of each center, the responsible person, and patient. The discontinuation of heparin infusion before cannula removal is also implemented differently depending on each center and the responsible person. Careful patient selection for the hemostasis method used and a proper method are needed for successful hemostasis following ECMO decannulation.

3.1 Manual or mechanical compression

All venous cannulas can be removed using a simple aseptic method. The operator must be aware of the danger of air embolism. This situation can be prevented by the application of Valsalva maneuver. The area around the venous cannula should be infiltrated with local anesthetic, and a horizontal mattress suture can be helpful to the hemostasis.

For percutaneous ECMO establishment, the artery was manually compressed after decannulation for 30–60 minutes. In case of persistent bleeding, a surgical correction was done. In the absence of any bleeding, only a standard pressure bandage or mechanical compressor was applied.

For a more definite hemostasis, prior to manual compression, if possible, modifiable coagulopathy factors such as activated coagulation time (ACT), activated partial thromboplastin time (aPTT), prothrombin time (PT), and platelet activation should be corrected. Yeo et al. reported the use of dual antiplatelet drugs and a higher aPTT can lead to an increased risk of postprocedural vascular complications. Therefore, manual compression should be applied cautiously after the correction of coagulopathy factors such as ACT, aPTT, and platelets counts [12].

Manual compression does not require movement of the patient and can be performed relatively easily without any special device. However, it may be difficult to obtain consistent results using this method, depending on the person applying compression. If a large cannula is used, the patient has severe calcification of the blood vessels, or long ECMO duration, is obese, or coagulopathy is not well corrected, it would be better to consider other methods. Further studies are necessary to evaluate the efficacy and safety of manual or mechanical compression in patients with ECMO.

3.2 Surgical repair

Peripheral or central cannulas inserted surgically should be removed surgically. If the arterial thrombosis was detected before ECMO weaning, the thrombosis can be removed together with surgical cannula removal.

Surgical removal has the advantage of visualizing blood vessels directly, removing the cannula, and stopping bleeding. Surgical removal can cause problems such as infection or poor healing of the wound and bleeding or lymphatic leakage. There is also a limitation in that it is possible only when a patient is moved to an operating room and surgical equipment is moved, or an operator is required.

Although more research is needed, surgical removal is thought to reduce the side effects if applied when large cannula is used, ECMO application period is long, and vascular calcification is severe.

3.3 The vascular closure device

In an effort to reduce the rates of vascular complications at the time of VA-ECMO decannulation and avoid the need for traditional surgical vascular repair, percutaneous techniques for closure of arterial cannulation sites utilizing several vascular closure systems have been employed by a number of centers [13].

Chandel et al. reported the use of a pre-closure technique was associated with a significant decrease in limb complications and bleeding events with an estimated 81% and 79% decreased likelihood of these complications, respectively, compared with surgical removal [13]. Data from prior cohorts have documented the utility of this technique in the removal of arterial sheaths of sizes ranging from 5 Fr to 24 Fr [13]. The main benefit of using this technique is the avoidance of a groin incision, which may be susceptible to wound infection, poor healing, and lymph leakage [14]. The procedure time is shorter than that of other methods.

This method also has disadvantages such as technical failure, thromboembolism, pseudoaneurysm, and stenosis, and is more expensive than other methods. If hemostasis is difficult or has failed, manual compression must be applied or conversion to surgery must be undertaken, which may cause a large amount of bleeding. After applying a closure device, it is necessary to closely monitor the occurrence of complications.

Some centers use closure devices for distal perfusion catheter removal [14].

However, as experience is accumulated with this technique, it may be possible to accomplish arterial ECMO decannulation at the bedside without the use of general anesthesia.

4. Conclusion

VA ECMO is an influential life support tool. Weaning from VA ECMO remains a challenging decision. In addition to cardiac function, overall patient evaluation should be done accurately to achieve successful ECMO weaning. It is especially important that the ECMO is not weaned while the patient is still recovering from the conditions that required the VA ECMO implantation.

Weaning strategies are based on institutional standards and individual experiences. Different weaning algorithms are used and none have reached dominance yet. Experienced VA ECMO centers should elaborate standardized weaning algorithms and consensus documents. A systematic weaning protocol will be able to lower the weaning failure rate.

Cannula removal should be selected well according to the patient's condition and the experience of the centers. It is also important to reduce complications by closely observing the patient after cannula removal.

Larger randomized trials are needed to confirm our findings and generate a new standard for VA-ECMO decannulation.

Acknowledgements

Thanks go to Asan Medical Center for having the experience and knowledge of ECMO.

Conflict of interest

The authors declare no conflict of interest.

Author details

Pilje Kang
Asan Medical Center, Seoul, Republic of Korea

*Address all correspondence to: kfeelj78@gmail.com

References

[1] Brogen TV, Lequier L, Lorusso R, MacLaren G, Peek G. Extracorporeal Life Support: The ELSO Red Book. 5th ed. Ann Arbor: Extracorporeal Support Organization; 2017

[2] Trahanas JM et al. How to turn it down: The evidence and opinions behind adult venoarterial extracorporeal membrane oxygenation weaning. ASAIO Journal. 2021;**67**(9):964-972

[3] Ortuno S et al. Weaning from veno-arterial extra-corporeal membrane oxygenation: Which strategy to use? Annals of Cardiothoracic Surgery. 2019;**8**(1):E1-E8

[4] Lusebrink E et al. Update on weaning from veno-arterial extracorporeal membrane oxygenation. Journal of Clinical Medicine. 2020;**9**(4):992

[5] Tohme J et al. Weaning-related shock in patients with ECMO: Incidence, mortality, and predisposing factors. Journal of Cardiothoracic and Vascular Anesthesia. 2021;**35**(1):41-47

[6] Hussey PT et al. Echocardiography for extracorporeal membrane oxygenation. Echocardiography. 2022;**39**(2):339-370

[7] Sawada K et al. Predicting parameters for successful weaning from Veno-arterial extracorporeal membrane oxygenation in cardiogenic shock. ESC Heart Failure. 2021;**8**(1):471-480

[8] Ling L, Chan KM. Weaning adult patients with cardiogenic shock on veno-arterial extracorporeal membrane oxygenation by pump-controlled retrograde trial off. Perfusion. 2018;**33**(5):339-345

[9] Pandya NR et al. A comparison of pump-controlled retrograde trial off to arterio-venous bridging for weaning from venoarterial extracorporeal membrane oxygenation. European Journal of Cardio-Thoracic Surgery. 2019;**56**:277-284

[10] Ju MH et al. Early experience of pump-controlled retrograde trial off for weaning from veno-arterial extracorporeal membrane oxygenation in adult patients with cardiogenic shock. Perfusion. 2021;**36**(4):401-406

[11] Heller S et al. Puncture and wiring of extracorporeal circuit for cannula safe removal or exchange. Perfusion. 2016;**31**(7):604-607

[12] Yeo HJ et al. Vascular complications arising from hemostasis with manual compression following extracorporeal membrane oxygenation decannulation. Journal of Cardiac Surgery. 2016;**31**(2):123-126

[13] Chandel A et al. Preclosure technique versus arterial cutdown after percutaneous cannulation for venoarterial extracorporeal membrane oxygenation. JTCVS Techniques. 2021;**10**:322-330

[14] Shah A et al. Complete percutaneous decannulation from femoral venoarterial extracorporeal membrane oxygenation. JTCVS Techniques. 2021;**6**:75-81

Chapter 8

ECMO for Respiratory Failure in the Patient with Advance Lung Disease: A Bridge to Recovery or Decision

Maria M. Crespo and Christian A. Bermudez

Abstract

Extracorporeal membrane oxygenation (ECMO) has clear benefits in patients with acute cardiopulmonary failure. However, selecting patients who will benefit from extracorporeal membrane oxygenation can be a challenge and remains a hurdle for clinicians today. An increased concern when considering ECMO therapy is whether the patient will recover enough function and be able to be weaned from ECMO support and survive to discharge or undergo lung transplantation and specially on whether to extend extracorporeal membrane oxygenation as a bridge to recovery in those with concerns of a meaningful recovery or as a bridge-to-decision (BTD) for patients whose criteria for lung transplantation are unknown. In addition, ECMO is a resource-intensive form of lung support that requires significant institutional commitment and a well-trained team to ensure good outcomes. The critical factors in the decision-making process when there are concerns regarding the initiation, continuation, or withdrawal of ECMO include early transfer to a specialized lung transplant center and a multidisciplinary consensus among lung transplant pulmonologists, lung transplant surgeons, and ECMO critical care intensivists to expedited transplant evaluation and to clearly defined the goals of care and selecting the appropriate candidates who will benefit from ECMO as a BTD for patients not listed yet for lung transplantation.

Keywords: ECMO, lung transplantation, indications, timing, patient selection, outcomes

1. Introduction

Since the 1950s, extracorporeal lung support has experienced continuous advancements in technology and a better understanding of ECMO physiology, which has led to less morbidity and more liberal use of this technology in acute respiratory failure (ARF). Experiences in selecting and managing patients with acute cardiac and respiratory failure treated with ECMO continue to grow. ECMO is a resource-intense form of lung support that requires significant institutional commitments and a well-trained team to ensure good outcomes.

There are clear benefits of ECMO in patients with acute respiratory failure such as acute respiratory distress syndrome (ARDS), hypercapneic respiratory failure related to infections or flare of their underlying disease, and pulmonary arterial hypertension (PAH) patients with decompensated right heart failure as a bridge-to-recovery (BTR), and as a bridge-to-decision (BTD) for lung transplant candidates, who have not completed the lung transplant evaluation, and as a bridge-to-transplant (BTT) for decompensated lung transplant candidates, hoping to avoid mechanical ventilation, sedation, and the use of neuromuscular blocking agents for conditioning, preservation of lung transplant candidacy, and ultimately better long-term outcomes. However, the decision to support patients with acute or acute-on-chronic respiratory failure with ECMO is challenging. No single guideline exists to aid decision-making, and the clinical management decisions are highly center-specific.

Based on the organ procurement and transplantation network (OPTN)/and the scientific registry of transplant recipient database (SRTR) 2020 report, lung transplant candidates hospitalized in the intensive care unit (ICU) comprised 13.8% of transplant recipients; 9.2% were hospitalized but not in the ICU. Also, candidates continued to be bridged-to-transplant; 3.6% on mechanical ventilation and ECMO, 1.8% on mechanical ventilation only, and 3.1% ECMO only [1].

This chapter will review the ECMO support as a BTR and as a BTD in patients with advanced lung disease and respiratory failure not listed for a lung transplant, including the limited data and the lack of good guidelines on candidate selection and the need for advance care planning, early palliative care involvement, and the need to involve patient and family on the implications of ECMO withdrawn when not a candidate for lung transplantation before deciding to accept ECMO as a bridge-to-decision.

2. ECMO as a bridge to recovery for acute respiratory failure in patients with advance lung disease

Treating patients with interstitial lung disease (ILD) and acute respiratory failure (ARF) is challenging. Lung transplantation is the only definitive therapy for patients with severe and meaningful recovery. Unfortunately, acute exacerbation of idiopathic pulmonary fibrosis (AE-IPF) is an often deadly complication of idiopathic pulmonary fibrosis (IPF).

Mechanical ventilation is a significant problem in advanced interstitial lung disease patients as the lung parenchyma is susceptible to ventilator-induced lung injury and oxygen toxicity [2, 3]. This likely triggers further disease progression [4]. Also, these patients often have secondary pulmonary hypertension and right ventricular dysfunction, increasing ventilation strategies' challenges [5]. Patients with advanced lung disease who developed respiratory failure and required mechanical ventilation have high mortality (70–90%) [6]. On the other hand, ECMO support might prevent ventilator-induced lung injury and worsening right ventricular dysfunction. However, the value of ECMO in patients with acute respiratory failure due to underlying lung fibrosis has not yet been well studied.

Kreuter *et al.* [7] published an international survey from 66 countries and 509 pulmonologists to assess the global variability in the prevention, diagnostic, and treatment of AE-IPF and reported that in case of respiratory failure, invasive ventilation was offered only to 45% to patients suitable for lung transplantation (LTx), as a BTT or in very selected other cases. Extracorporeal membrane oxygenation was offered to 44% of patients suitable for LTx as a bridge-to-transplant, mainly in Europe (57%) and the fewest in Oceania (24%). Palliative care was considered by 65% of the pulmonologist. The differences in these approaches were again significant between continents. Some of the differences in approaches might be related to center protocols, ICU resources, and ECMO expertise team experiences. Technology and resources also vary among countries.

2.1 ECMO for acute respiratory distress syndrome

Several landmark trials of venovenous (VV)—ECMO for acute respiratory distress syndrome (ARDS) are often referenced when discussing the potential benefits of ECMO for respiratory failure. Key studies supporting the efficacy of ECMO include the Australian and New Zealand study on H1N1-induced ARDS patients treated with ECMO having greater than 70% survival [8]. Around this time, major improvements were made to the ECMO devices, including more efficient oxygenators, fewer thrombotic centrifugal pumps, and improved percutaneous vascular access cannulas.

Peek *et al.* [9] conducted a multicenter randomized control trial based in the UK called the CESAR trial, where patients with ARDS were randomized to conventional therapy or ECMO, showing that patients with ARDS who were referred to an ECMO center had significantly improved survival 6 months from discharge than those who were not referred and treated with medical management alone. Severe ARDS was defined as a Murray score above three or an arterial pH below 7.20. Essential exclusion criteria were prolonged high oxygen requirement or high-pressure mechanical ventilation for more than 7 days before considering enrollment. The results of the CESAR trial showed improved survival without severe disability in the patients considered for ECMO. 63% of the ECMO consideration group was alive at 6 months, whereas only 47% of the conventional therapy group survived that timeframe. Most deaths in the ECMO group were from multi-system organ failure, whereas 60% of the standard therapy patients died of respiratory failure. The release of the data from the CESAR trial and the treatment successes from the 2009 Influenza pandemic has propagated ECMO use in various clinical settings.

The REVA study group published their results using ECMO for H1N1-associated ARDS and identified at 1-year post-ICU discharge that 83% of patients treated with ECMO had returned to work vs. 64% of non-ECMO treated patients [10].

The ECMO to Rescue Lung Injury in Severe ARDS (EOLIA) clinical trial randomized patients to VV ECMO based on blood gas and ventilator criteria similar to CESAR [11]. However, its results further clouded the data regarding the benefits of ECMO for refractory ARDS. In total, 249 patients were randomized in the study, and there were no significant differences between the two groups. At the primary endpoint of 60 days, 35% of the ECMO group had died, whereas 46% of the control group was dead. The highest sub-group mortality was those patients who crossed over from the control group to ECMO, as 57% of them were dead by 60-days. They concluded that among patients with very severe ARDS, 60-day mortality was not significantly lower with ECMO than with a strategy of conventional mechanical ventilation that included ECMO as rescue therapy. Despite what appears to be trending toward better survival with earlier ECMO, the data did not reach statistical significance.

2.2 ECMO for hypercapnic respiratory failure

The treatment of acute exacerbations of chronic obstructive lung disease (COPD) resulting in hypercapnic respiratory failure refractory to medical treatment has been invasive mechanical ventilation (IMV). In the most severe cases, these may be refractory to conventional therapies and mechanical ventilation, becoming life-threatening. Invasive mechanical ventilation develops a considerable reduction in respiratory muscle strength, having a higher risk of prolonged weaning and failure to wean compared to other causes of acute hypercapnic respiratory failure and a more increased need for early tracheostomy. These patients also have a higher risk of developing complications such as ventilator-associated pneumonia (VAP), ventilator-induced lung injury (VILI), ventilator-associated diaphragmatic dysfunction (VIDD), and critical illness myopathy and neuropathy associated with steroids and neuromuscular blockade agents often used during their critical ICU admission [12]. Extracorporeal carbon dioxide removal (ECCO2R) represents an attractive approach in this setting for carbon dioxide removal options to avoid and possibly prevent worsening respiratory failure and respiratory acidosis and shorten the duration of IMV.

In 2009, Dr. Zwischenberger's group successfully used venovenous-ECMO for carbon dioxide removal (ECCO2R) in a hypercarbic patient with COPD. They successfully reduced PaCO2, minute ventilation, and ventilator pressures [13]. In 2013, the Columbia University group used ECCO2R to facilitate extubation in five patients with COPD, all of whom had failed to wean from the ventilator. These patients were extubated in a median time of 4 h and most were ambulatory within 24 h of venovenous ECMO initiation. Once extubated, patients were rehabilitated while on ECCO2R, with a mean time to ambulation of 19.4 ± 12.6 hours after ECCO2R. Moreover, all patients survived hospital discharge [14]. Since that time, multiple reports have supported the efficacy of venovenous ECMO in treating hypercapnic respiratory failure in COPD and reducing intubation time or preventing it all together [15, 16]. In the ÉCLAIR study, Braune *et al.* [16] showed that IMV was avoided in 56% of cases treated with ECCO2R but was associated with a higher incidence of complications.

Although ECCO2R seems effective in improving or mitigating hypercapnic acidosis and possibly reducing the rate of endotracheal intubation, its use is associated with a range of vascular, hematological, and other complications. Thrombocytopenia and heparin-induced thrombocytopenia are also commonly observed. Other serious complications associated with arterial cannulation include distal limb ischemia, compartment syndrome of the lower limb requiring fasciotomy, or limb amputation [17]. Bleeding is the most common complication of ECCO2R. The need for anticoagulation increases the risk of significant bleeding, including cerebral, gastrointestinal, and nasopharyngeal bleeds. The published incidence of substantial bleeding complications is between 2 and 50% [18].

2.3 ECMO for pulmonary arterial hypertension

Patients with group 1 pulmonary arterial hypertension (PAH) and decompensated right ventricular failure (RHF) were not previously considered for ECMO as a BTT or BTR because options were limited by the idea that PAH patients would not be able to weaned from ECMO as a BTR from an acute decompensation and by long transplantation wait times and perceived inability to weaned from ECMO. Rosenzweig *et al.* [19] published a retrospective review of ECMO as a BTR for PAH. A total of six patients (age 32 ± 11 years) underwent ECMO bridging. Two patients who were considered good candidates for lung transplantation underwent successful ECMO-BTT. Four patients who were not regarded as promising candidates for lung transplantation experienced ECMO-BTR with the escalation of targeted medical therapies before weaning off ECMO. Three of four ECMO-BTR patients survived ECMO decannulation (duration 7–23 days). This single-institution experience demonstrated the beneficial use of upper body configuration ECMO strategy without mechanical support in PAH patients as a BTR or BTT when they failed to respond to medical therapy. In addition, this strategy facilitates mobility with physical therapy, thereby optimizing transplant candidacy.

Chicotka *et al.* [20] published a retrospective review of 50 patients with interstitial lung disease and pulmonary hypertension treated initially with either VV or veno-arterial (VA) ECMO as a bridge-to-transplant. They found that patients with early VA ECMO initiation had significantly better survival to transplantation than those with early VV ECMO ($p = 0.03$). In addition, there was a 59% reduction in risk of death for VA compared with VV ECMO (HR 0.41, 95% confidence interval: 0.18 to 0.92, $p = 0.03$) shown by cox proportional hazards modeling. Also, there was an 80% reduction in the risk of death when ambulating on ECMO before lung transplant (HR 20, 95% confidence interval: 0.08 to 0.48, $p < 0.01$). In this single-institution experience, they found that combined ECMO with targeted PAH therapies was successfully used as BTT or BTR for acute right heart failure in group 1 PAH patients leading to significant improvement in gas exchange and end-organ function. Unfortunately, only 10 patients in this series of 50 were IPAH and 5 Eisenmenger. This approach needs further assessment, and as experience grows, we may anticipate earlier instituting ECMO in suitable group 1 PAH patients.

3. ECMO as a bridge-to-decision or bridge-to-transplant in patients with advance lung disease

The most significant issue with lung transplantation is often long wait times. This problem seems more prominent in the Eurotransplant area than in the United Network for Organ Sharing area. Based on the OPTN/SRTR 2022 report, lung transplant candidates continued to be bridged-to-transplant; 3.6% on mechanical ventilation and ECMO, 1.8% on mechanical ventilation only, and 3.1% ECMO only and ECMO-BTT patients who survive to LTx have a post-transplant survival rate comparable to those who did not receive ECMO pre-transplant [1].

Traditionally, the concept of ECMO use in respiratory failure was to initiate it in conjunction with invasive mechanical ventilation and later by discontinuing ECMO support before ventilator weaning. However, with the ability of ECMO to take over the function of the gas exchange of the ventilator, this pattern is changing, and it will continue to evolve as further technological improvements are made. Some centers have reported successfully starting ECMO instead of invasive mechanical ventilation, bypassing the ventilator entirely [21, 22]. Abrams *et al.* [21] described an evolving paradigm of extracorporeal membrane oxygenation (ECMO) in respiratory failure as a temporary adjunct to invasive mechanical ventilation in severe respiratory failure and using ECMO to facilitate removal or avoidance of IMV while bridge-to-recovery or bridge-to-transplant, at their institution. The paradigm of bridge-to-transplant or bridge-to-decision from IMV and ECMO remains a consideration. However, it remains to be defined who are the specific patient populations for whom these strategies are most appropriate, including those with hypercapnic respiratory failure or awaiting lung transplantation.

Salna and Bacchetta [23] described a clinical decision-making algorithm used at their institution to optimize ECMO configurations and cannulation strategies based on patients' pathophysiology using a multidisciplinary ECMO team approach for BTT. Factors to decide whether patients will benefit from BTT were age, functional status on admission, underlying disease, infection or other organ system dysfunction, and anticipated waitlist time. The primary goal of using ECMO as a BTT was to optimize transplant candidates before transplantation to improve lung transplant outcomes. Their goal was to help ambulation, which depends on optimal cannulation configurations and early physiotherapy, with patients being mobilized as early as ECMO day 1 [24]. They also aim to cannulate patients without intubation or general anesthesia whenever possible for accelerated recovery or optimization for transplantation.

Trudzinski *et al.* [25] published a retrospective analysis of patients with ILD and ARF treated with or without ECMO from March 2012 to August 2015. Forty patients with interstitial lung disease referred to their intensive care unit for acute respiratory failure were included in the analysis. Twenty-one were treated with ECMO. ECMO was initiated regardless of whether they could be a lung transplant candidate. From the total of 13 patients who were evaluated, eight were found adequate candidates for ECMO as a BTT. Six patients underwent lung transplantation, and 14 of the 15 patients who did not undergo lung transplantation (93.3%) died after 40.3 ± 27.8 days on ECMO. 83.3% of the patients who had a lung transplant were able to be discharged from the hospital. Their important finding was that those patients with ILD on ECMO who were not lung transplant candidates had a high mortality rate, comparable with the mortality rate of patients mechanically ventilated. Also, they demonstrated that ECMO had no value as a transplant-independent outcome improvement in ILD. On the other hand, patients who are candidates for lung transplantation benefit from ECMO therapy. The biggest reason for this benefit is the time gained on ECMO. They concluded that ECMO is a lifesaving option for patients with ILD and ARF provided they are candidates for lung transplantation. Unfortunately, ECMO cannot reverse the poor prognosis in patients who do not qualify for lung transplantation.

Decision supporting patients with acute or acute-on-chronic respiratory failure with ECMO is challenging, and there is no single guideline to help in decision-making. Even so, several high-volume lung transplants and ECMO centers have published their experience with ECMO as a bridge to transplant [22, 26, 27]. A typical decision tree of ECMO as a bridge-to-transplant algorithmic implementation, used only for those listed patients, as shown in **Figure 1** (adapted from Biscotti *et al.* [26]).

The timing of ECMO implementation is crucial. Therefore, they attempted to select patients in whom post-ECMO rehabilitation is likely, as best predicted by patients' pre-ECMO physical therapy performance. The aim was to liberate all patients from mechanical ventilation by using strategies such as early tracheostomy. The criteria for initiating physical therapy included hemodynamic stability, secure cannulas without active bleeding, and patient willingness to cooperate. Ambulation was implemented once the patients demonstrated physiologically adequate ECMO support is demonstrated during initial bedside physical therapy. Seventy-two patients received ECMO as a bridge to LTx. Of the 72 patients, 55.6% underwent the transplantation procedure, 92.5% survived to discharge, and 84% survived for 2 years. Patients with cystic fibrosis were more likely to have a BTT than patients with other lung diseases. Daily participation in physical therapy was achieved in 69.4% of patients. This study demonstrated favorable survival in patients receiving ECMO as a BTT, attaining high rates of physical therapy, and avoiding mechanical ventilation in patients awaiting lung transplantation. With more than half of these patients successfully BTT, we gained insight into the factors influencing patients' outcomes, including patient selection, the timing of ECMO, and patient management. However, clinical management decisions are highly center-specific, and these treatment algorithms must be adapted to fit the clinical setting appropriately.

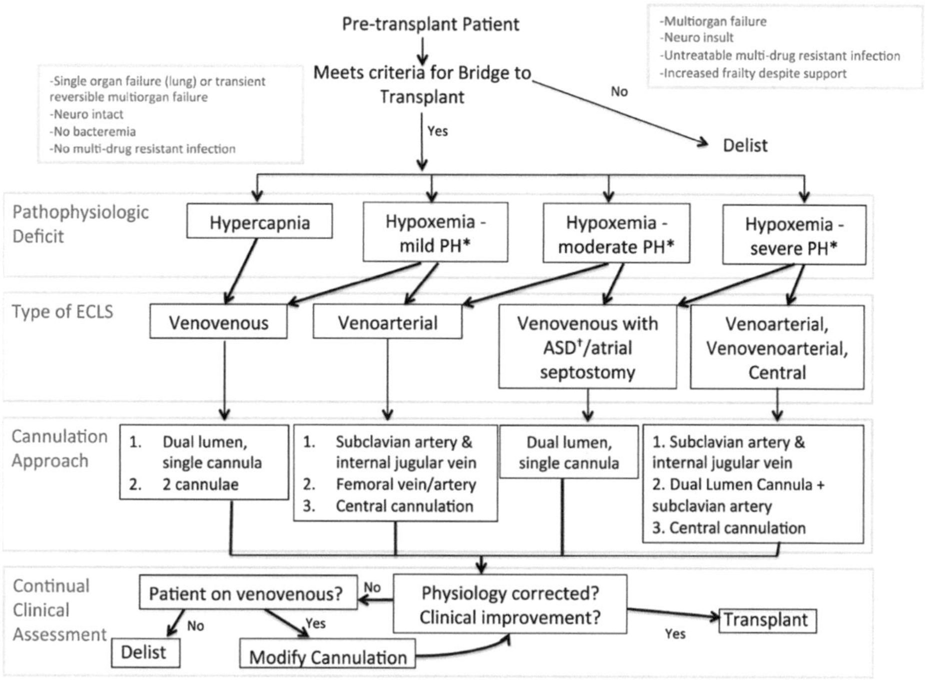

Figure 1.
*Bridge to transplantation decision algorithm. *Pulmonary hypertension (PH). †Atrial septal defect (ASD). (ECLS = extracorporeal life support). Adapted from Biscotti et al. [26].*

The cannulation strategy was based on the patient's underlying disease, respiratory and hemodynamic status, and anticipated worsening of hypoxemia or progressive secondary pulmonary hypertension (PH). They also attempt to select patients in whom post-ECMO rehabilitation is likely, as best predicted by patients' pre-ECMO physical therapy performance. The form of 'awake ECMO' with spontaneously breathing patients is a safe and effective approach to BTT [26–29]. Several high-volume centers have shown that BTT has comparable outcomes with patients not requiring support [26, 27, 30–32].

Another meaningful discussion is the outcomes in the unique subset of patients requiring prolonged use of ECMO support before lung transplantation. In a 2016 review of the Extracorporeal Life Support Organization international multi-institutional registry, of 974 patients who required prolonged (>14 days) ECMO support, 46% of these patients did not experience native lung recovery; among these, 40 patients (4.1%) underwent LTx with a 50% postoperative in-hospital mortality [33]. The longest reported successful bridge to transplant required ECMO support of 155 days [34]. Another case report describes a patient remaining on ECMO for as long as 403 days while waiting for a lung transplant. The authors conclude that it is at least technically feasible to maintain patients awaiting lung transplantation on ECMO for extended periods, albeit maintaining for more than 1-year may be difficult [35]. ECMO cannot reverse the poor prognosis in patients that do not qualify for lung transplantation. ARF in ILD is devastating in patients without the option of a lung transplant, despite ECMO.

The current biggest challenges for clinicians are when to consider ECMO as a BTD in patients with end-stage lung disease not yet listed for lung transplantation. The decision is less about using ECMO-BTT and more about whether to extend ECMO-BTD to patients whose lung transplant candidate status is unknown and whether the patient clinically deteriorates while completing their lung transplant evaluation. Also, what if ECMO is needed to facilitate a remaining component of the transplant workup if a previously healthy patient has failed all interventions following an acute, irreversible pulmonary disease. Hoopes and colleagues [22] described a salvage transplant as a feasible approach in this cohort. Although the precise relationship between providing ECMO to patients before active listing and survival to transplant is unknown, their study examined 31 patients who successfully had ECMO-BTT, including seven patients not yet listed for transplant prior to ECMO initiation. The 1-year outcomes of the patients transplanted from an ECMO-BTT was greater than 90% [22]. In this context, rescue therapy denotes lung transplantation in patients not listed before ARF. In particular, salvage transplantation opens a window for clinically sick patients who are not yet listed for lung transplantation, allowing them to be transferred on ECMO to a facility and have an expedited evaluation for potential lung transplantation.

Patients with ILD that survived mechanical ventilation to discharge had a very limited prognosis without lung transplantation; 1-year survival rates were only 4% [36]. In some situations, such as acute exacerbation of ILD, it may be preferable to initiate ECMO-BTD, avoid intubation and mechanical ventilation, the use of sedation helping being awake, maintenance in the nutrition status, mobilization avoiding frailty, and provide emotional support for the patient and the family, and allowing patients who are otherwise considered good candidates to be able to complete the lung transplant evaluation.

Ideally, the bridge-to-decision patients have been already evaluated for a lung transplant and are hospitalized at an expertise lung transplant and ECMO center with adequate ICU resources to support these complex patients with the potential for long-term care, and the patient has completed part of the key initial lung transplant evaluation so that the remaining of the completed evaluation can be expedited, and that the patient does not have any obvious contraindications to be a candidate for lung transplantation.

In general, bridge-to-decision patients should have minimal or absent characteristics that have been associated with worse bridge-to-transplant survival. A multidisciplinary consensus among the lung transplant physicians, critical care intensivists, and ECMO team is essential for a successful transition from ECMO-BTD to ECMO-BTT. in addition, daily multidisciplinary rounds, including advanced care planning and early palliative care involvement are important. The patient and their family should be encouraged to reflect on these implications before deciding to accept ECMO bridge-to-decision. The decision to provide ECMO to patients with advanced lung disease not yet listed for lung transplant should apply existing data and expert opinion to the clinical circumstance. With tempered judgment and expert care, ECMO can provide a pathway to life for patients with end-stage lung disease who are not listed for a lung transplant at the time of their critical admission.

Another concern is when patients, who have started ECMO support, are not candidates for LTx. This situation is ethically challenging and emotionally charged, referred to as a 'bridge to nowhere“, with obvious implications for the patient, their family, the caregivers, the hospital, and the healthcare system" [37]. Therefore, it is important to minimize this risk as much as possible through meticulous patient selection. Other concerns for decisions on considering patients who are candidates for ECMO BTD are those patients who are highly sensitized and have a higher risk for worsening sensitization due to ECMO-related needs for blood transfusion and concerns for increased waiting times, infections risk, and vascular complications. Other concerns for decisions on considering patients who are candidates for ECMO BTD are those patients who are highly sensitized and have higher risk for worsening sensitization due to ECMO related need for blood transfusion and concerns for increase waiting times, infections risk and vascular complications.

Even though ECMO as a BTD can benefit patients and families by giving them more time to share with each other and for discussions on collaborative decision-making. Courtwright *et al.* states the most common ethical issues involving disagreements among and between healthcare teams, patients, family, and other surrogates, particularly when confronted with decisions about the continuation or withdrawal of ECMO [38].

4. Conclusions

ECMO is a lifesaving option for patients with advanced lung disease, and ARF provided they are suitable candidates for lung transplantation. Salvage transplantation opens a door for clinically sick patients who are not yet listed for lung transplantation, allowing them to be transferred on ECMO to a facility and have an expedited evaluation for potential lung transplantation. There is limited data and a lack of good guidelines on candidate selection.

The question regarding using ECMO as a BTD in patients with end-stage lung disease not yet listed for lung transplantation and if the patient clinically deteriorates while nearing completion of their transplant evaluation, or if ECMO support is needed to facilitate completing the lung transplant evaluation, is more challenged than whether using ECMO-BTT.

Daily interdisciplinary rounds, advanced care planning, and early palliative care involvement are essential. The patient and family should be encouraged to reflect on these implications before deciding to accept ECMO-BTD. It is important to have a protocol for ECMO withdrawal when not a candidate for LTx. Consensus guidelines on ECMO-BTD for patients, not jet listed for LTx as risk stratification to better assess those patients who will benefit the most and have the best outcomes post-transplant.

Author details

Maria M. Crespo[1]* and Christian A. Bermudez[2]

1 Division of Pulmonary, Allergy, and Critical Care, Hospital of the University of Pennsylvania, Philadelphia, Pennsylvania, USA

2 Division of Cardiac Surgery, Hospital of the University of Pennsylvania, Philadelphia, Pennsylvania, USA

*Address all correspondence to: maria.crespo@pennmedicine.upenn.edu

References

[1] Valapour M, Lehr CJ, Skeans MA, Smith JM, et al. OPTN/SRTR 2020. Annual Data Report: Lung. American Journal of Transplantation. 2022;**22**(2):432-518. DOI: 10.1111/ajt.16991

[2] Rachmale S, Li G, Wilson G, Malinchoc M, Gajic O. Practice of excessive F(IO(2)) and effect on pulmonary outcomes in mechanically ventilated patients with acute lung injury. Respiratory Care. 2012;**57**:1887-1893

[3] Anzueto S, Frutos-Vivar F, Esteban A, Alia I, Brochard L, Stewart T, et al. Incidence, risk factors and outcomes of barotrauma in mechanical ventilated patients. Intensive Care Medicine. 2004;**30**:612-619

[4] Martin TR, Nakamura M, Matute-Bello G. The role of apoptosis in acute lung injury. Critical Care Medicine. 2003;**31**(Suppl. 4):S184-S188

[5] Nakos G, Tsangaris I, Kostanti E, Nathanail C, Lachana A, Koulouras V, et al. Effect of the prone position on patients with hydrostatic pulmonary edema compared with patients with acute respiratory distress syndrome and pulmonary fibrosis. American Journal of Respiratory and Critical Care Medicine. 2000;**161**:360-368

[6] Fumeaux T, Rothmeier C, Jolliet P. Outcome of mechanical ventilation for acute respiratory failure in patients with pulmonary fibrosis. Intensive Care Medicine. 2001;**27**:1868-1874

[7] Kreuter M, Polke M, Simon IF, et al. Acute exacerbation of idiopathic pulmonary fibrosis: International survey and call for harmonization. European Respiratory Journal. 2020;**55**:1901760. DOI: 10.1183/13993003.01760-2019

[8] Webb SA, Pettila V, Seppelt I, et al. Critical care services and 2009 H1N1 influenza in Australia and New Zealand. The New England Journal of Medicine. 2009;**361**:1925-1934

[9] Peek GJ, Mugford M, Tiruvoipati R, et al. Efficacy and economic assessment of conventional ventilatory support versus extracorporeal membrane oxygenation for severe adult respiratory failure (CESAR): A multicenter randomized controlled trial. Lancet. 2009;**374**:1351-1363

[10] Luyt CE, Combes A, Becquemin MH, et al. Long-term outcomes of pandemic 2009 influenza a(H1N1)-associated severe ARDS. Chest. 2012;**142**:583-592

[11] Combes A, Hajage G, Capellier G, et al. Extracorporeal membrane oxygenation for severe acute respiratory distress syndrome. The New England Journal of Medicine. 2018;**378**(21):1965-1975

[12] Nava S, Ambrosino N, Clini E, Prato M, Orlando G, Vitacca M, et al. Noninvasive mechanical ventilation in the weaning of patients with respiratory failure due to chronic obstructive pulmonary disease. A randomized, controlled trial. Annals of Internal Medicine. 1998;**128**(9):721-728

[13] Cardenas VJ Jr, Lynch JE, Ates R, Miller L, Zwischenberger JB. Venovenous carbon dioxide removal in chronic obstructive pulmonary disease: Experience in one patient. ASAIO Journal. 2009;**55**(4):420-422. DOI: 10.1097/MAT.0b013e3181a7b55d

[14] Abrams DC, Brenner K, Burkart KM, et al. Pilot study of extracorporeal carbon dioxide removal to facilitate extubation and ambulation in exacerbations of chronic obstructive pulmonary disease.

Annals of the American Thoracic Society. 2013;**10**:307-314

[15] Kluge S, Braune SA, Engel M, et al. Avoiding invasive mechanical ventilation by extracorporeal carbon dioxide removal in patients failing noninvasive ventilation. Intensive Care Medicine. 2012;**38**:1632-1639

[16] Braune S, Sieweke A, Brettner F, et al. The feasibility and safety of extracorporeal carbon dioxide removal to avoid intubation in patients with COPD unresponsive to noninvasive ventilation for acute hypercapnic respiratory failure (ECLAIR study): Multicentre case-control study. Intensive Care Medicine. 2016;**42**:1437-1444

[17] Cove ME, MacLaren G, Federspiel WJ, Kellum JA. Bench to bedside review: Extracorporeal carbon dioxide removal, past present and future. Critical Care. 2012;**16**(5):232

[18] Sklar MC, Beloncle F, Katsios CM, Brochard L, Friedrich JO. Extracorporeal carbon dioxide removal in patients with chronic obstructive pulmonary disease: A systematic review. Intensive Care Medicine. 2015;**41**:1752-1762. DOI: 10.1007/s00134-015-3921-z

[19] Rosenzweig EB, Brodie D, Abrams DC, Agerstrand CL, Bacchetta M. Extracorporeal membrane oxygenation as a novel bridging strategy for acute right heart failure in group 1 pulmonary arterial hypertension. SAIO Journal. 2014;**60**(1):129-133. DOI: 10.1097/MAT.0000000000000021

[20] Chicotka S, Pedroso FE, Agerstrand CL, Rosenzweig EB, Abrams D, et al. Increasing opportunity for lung transplant in interstitial lung disease with pulmonary hypertension. The Annals of Thoracic Surgery. 2018;**106**(6):1812-1819

[21] Abrams D, Brodie D. Emerging indications for extracorporeal membrane oxygenation in adults with respiratory failure. Annals ATS. 2013;**10**(4):371-377. DOI: 10.1513/AnnalsATS.201305-113OT

[22] Hoopes CW, Kukreja J, Golden J, Davenport DL, Diaz-Guzman E, Zwischenberger JB. Extracorporeal membrane oxygenation as a bridge to pulmonary transplantation. The Journal of Thoracic and Cardiovascular Surgery. 2013;**145**(3):862-868

[23] Salna M, Bacchetta M. Extracorporeal lung support. Current Opinion in Anesthesiology. 2017;**30**(1):50-57. DOI: 10.1097/ACO.0000000000000415

[24] Biscotti M, Bacchetta M. The "sport model": Extracorporeal membrane oxygenation using the subclavian artery. The Annals of Thoracic Surgery. 2014;**98**:1487-1489

[25] Trudzinski FC, Kaestner F, Schäfers H-J, et al. Outcome of Patients with Interstitial Lung Disease Treated with Extracorporeal Membrane Oxygenation for Acute Respiratory Failure: American Journal of Respiratory and Critical Care Medicine. 2015;**193**(5):527-533. DOI: 10.1164/rccm.201508-1701OC

[26] Biscotti M, Gannon WD, Agerstrand C, Abrams D, Sonett J, Brodie D, et al. Awake extracorporeal membrane oxygenation as bridge to lung transplantation: A 9-year experience. The Annals of Thoracic Surgery. 2017;**104**(2):412-419

[27] Biscotti M, Sonett J, Bacchetta M. ECMO as bridge to lung transplant. Thoracic Surgery Clinics. 2015;**25**:17-25

[28] Abrams DC, Brodie D, Rosenzweig EB, et al. Upper-body extracorporeal

membrane oxygenation as a strategy in decompensated pulmonary arterial hypertension. Pulmonary Circulation. 2013;**3**:432-435

[29] Biscotti M, Vail E, Cook KE, et al. Extracorporeal membrane oxygenation using subclavian artery cannulation in awake patients with pulmonary hypertension. ASAIO Journal. 2014;**60**:748-750

[30] Javidfar J, Brodie D, Wang D, Ibrahimiye AN, Yang J, Zwischenberger JB, et al. Use of bicaval dual-lumen catheter for adult venovenous extracorporeal membrane oxygenation. The Annals of Thoracic Surgery. 2011;**91**(6):1763-1769

[31] Toyoda Y, Bhama JK, Shigemura N, Zaldonis D, Pilewski J, Crespo M, et al. Efficacy of extracorporeal membrane oxygenation as a bridge to lung transplantation. The Journal of Thoracic and Cardiovascular Surgery. 2013;**145**(4):1065-1071

[32] Bermudez CA, Rocha RV, Zaldonis D, Bhama JK, Crespo MM, et al. Extracorporeal membrane oxygenation as a bridge to lung transplant; midterm outcomes. The Annals of Thoracic Surgery. 2011;**92**:1226-1231

[33] Posluszny J, Rycus PT, Bartlett RH, Engoren M, Haft JW, Lynch WR, et al. Outcome of adult respiratory failure patients receiving prolonged (≥14 days) ECMO. Annals of Surgery. 2016;**263**(3):573-581

[34] Kon ZN, Wehman PB, Gibber M, et al. Venovenous extracorporeal membrane oxygenation as a bridge to lung transplantation: Successful transplantation after 155 days of support. The Annals of Thoracic Surgery. 2015;**99**(2):704-707. DOI: 10.1016/j.athoracsur.2014.04.097

[35] Umei N, Ichiba S, Sakamoto A. Idiopathic pulmonary fibrosis patient supported with extracorporeal membrane oxygenation for 403 days while waiting for a lung transplant: A case report. Respiratory Medicine Case Reports. 2018;**24**:86-88

[36] Gaudry S, Vincent F, Rabbat A, Nunes H, Crestani B, Naccache JM, et al. Invasive mechanical ventilation in patients with fibrosing interstitial pneumonia. The Journal of Thoracic and Cardiovascular Surgery. 2014;**147**:47-53

[37] Abrams DC, Prager K, Blinderman CD, Burkart KM, Brodie D. Ethical dilemmas encountered with the use of extracorporeal membrane oxygen in adults. Chest. 2014;**145**(4):876-882

[38] Courtwright AM, Robinson EM, Feins K, et al. Ethics committee consultation and extracorporeal membrane oxygenation. Annals of the American Thoracic Society. 2016;**13**:1553-1558

Chapter 9

The Utility of ECMO in Acute Respiratory Distress Syndrome

Ashley K. Binder and Sunit Singla

Abstract

The state of knowledge regarding the adverse effects of mechanical ventilation in severe acute respiratory distress syndrome (ARDS) will be reviewed along with the benefits and limitations of lung protective ventilation strategies such as low tidal volume ventilation, prone positioning, and neuromuscular blockade. The potential for the use of ECMO as an ARDS-specific lung protective strategy, particularly as technology and experience at major medical centers advances, will be discussed. Experiences with the use of ECMO for ARDS during the COVID pandemic will be highlighted. Current accepted indications for ECMO in ARDS, based on published guidelines and trial data, will be examined. Finally, predictions about future directions for research in this area will be offered.

Keywords: acute respiratory distress syndrome, refractory hypoxemia, hypoxia, respiratory failure, hypoxic respiratory failure, extracorporeal membrane oxygenation, mechanical ventilation

1. Introduction

Acute respiratory distress syndrome (ARDS) consists of multiple underlying disease pathways and patterns of lung injury. When these progress to acute critical illness, all converge on the development of non-cardiogenic pulmonary edema [1]. CT chest imaging studies of ARDS patients have revealed that the amount of inflammatory pulmonary edema fluid correlates with gravity-dependent alveolar collapse [2, 3]. The sterno-vertebral distribution of aeration versus alveolar collapse during ARDS is the key to understanding the mechanisms of lung protective ventilatory strategies including low tidal volume ventilation, prone positioning, neuromuscular blockade, and, in the most severe cases, extracorporeal membrane oxygenation (ECMO).

2. Low tidal volume ventilation (LTVV)

The first of these, low tidal volume ventilation (LTVV), has remained the mainstay of recommended management strategies for ARDS for the past two decades as a result of clear mortality benefits elicited in randomized controlled studies [4]. It is based on the idea that the functional amount of aerated lung available to participate in tidal ventilation during ARDS is much smaller than normal [5], and that the potential detrimental effects of permissive hypercapnic acidosis (to a certain extent) are outweighed by the prevention of alveolar stretch-mediated injury during mechanical ventilation. While the ideal tidal volume for any given individual patient remains a matter of debate, the principle of lung protection from excessive tidal volume-induced lung injury, with its consequent reduction in mortality, has been confirmed by meta-analyses of multiple randomized controlled trials as well as two prospective cohort studies [3, 6–8]. Conversely, poor adherence to LTVV in ARDS has been prospectively associated with worse mortality [6, 7].

As pulmonary edema fluid increases, progressive de-recruitment of alveolar gas-exchanging units occurs. In moderate to severe forms of ARDS, the degree of de-recruitment may be so severe that even the delivery of 100% oxygen is insufficient to maintain an acceptable level of hemoglobin oxygen saturation/oxygen delivery for a critically ill patient. Additional reasons to avoid high amounts of oxygen include the potential for increased generation of reactive oxygen species resulting in increased tissue injury [9]. In these circumstances, it becomes necessary to recruit collapsed alveolar units to participate in gas exchange via the application of positive end-expiratory pressure (PEEP). Depending on the severity of gas exchange impairment, the application of PEEP typically ranges between 8 and 20 cm H_2O. However, when oxygenation is acutely and dangerously low, typically shortly after induction and intubation of a severe ARDS patient, high amounts of PEEP (up to 45 cm H_2O known as a recruitment maneuver) are sometimes temporarily applied for short periods of time to emergently recruit collapsed alveolar units. It should be noted that the routine, non-judicious application of recruitment maneuvers has been shown to increase mortality in ARDS patients [10], and therefore it is reserved only for emergent, salvage situations.

The reason for this lies in the observed heterogeneity of PEEP-responsiveness amongst ARDS patients. CT chest imaging studies have identified groups of patients who demonstrate near-immediate anatomic recruitment of collapsed alveolar units after the application of PEEP versus those who require longer periods of time or who do not exhibit any appreciable anatomic recruitment following a recruitment maneuver and/or increases in applied PEEP [11, 12]. Patients who fall closer to this latter group along the spectrum of PEEP-responsiveness are susceptible during PEEP application to alveolar overdistension in well-aerated regions of the lung (with resultant stretch-mediated injury) [12] as well as hemodynamic compromise resulting from an imposition on ventricular preload [13]. Furthermore, the excessive application of PEEP out of proportion to the degree of responsiveness in any given patient may result in functional decruitment due to decreasing perfusion of aerated alveoli.

Prone positioning is utilized to manage patients with relatively low levels of PEEP responsiveness. It reduces the recruitment threshold by reducing the compressive effects of the heart and abdomen as well as by causing more even pleural pressure distribution [14, 15]. The contribution of PEEP non-responsiveness to alveolar overinflation and augmentation of lung injury is demonstrated by significant decreases in mortality with the use of prone positioning in severe ARDS across multiple studies [16–23].

Non-homogenous distribution of pleural pressures during severe ARDS also contributes to the development of the injurious phenomenon of "pendelluft" or "swinging air" during spontaneous breathing efforts occurring while ARDS patients are deeply sedated but not paralyzed on mechanical ventilation [24]. This leads to overstretch of dependent aerated lung during early inflation with air moving to these regions without a change in tidal volume. However, the contribution of pendelluft to the perpetuation of lung injury during severe ARDS is currently unclear, as data from two large randomized controlled studies examining the use of neuromuscular blockade are conflicting with regards to a mortality benefit attributable to this management strategy [25, 26].

Much of the work done to improve clinical management and outcomes in ARDS patients has validated the concept of abrogating further injury by lung protective measures. Despite many advances along these lines, mortality from ARDS remains high [27], particularly in very severe cases where extreme levels of acidosis and hypoxemia limit the safe applicability of lung protective strategies. It is within this niche that a role for extracorporeal support has developed, which allows substantial, additional lung protection in extreme circumstances via a marked reduction in intrinsic gas exchange requirements. The injured lung can therefore be rested and allowed to recover without further exacerbation.

3. Studies

Three studies, two major randomized controlled trials and one matched paired analysis [28–30], have evaluated the use of ECMO in the clinical care of severe ARDS patients. The Conventional ventilatory support versus Extracorporeal membrane oxygenation for Severe Acute Respiratory failure (CESAR) trial studied 180 patients with severe acute respiratory failure who were randomly assigned either to be referred to a single ECMO center in the UK or to undergo continued conventional management as outlined above [28]. Severe respiratory failure was defined by the presence of one out of two criteria. The first was hypercapnic respiratory acidosis with a pH < 7.20 which would limit allowance of further permissive hypercapnia via lung protective ventilatory strategies. The second used the Murray lung injury score which is based on the ratio of arterial oxygen tension to the fraction of inspired oxygen (PaO_2/FiO_2), PEEP, lung compliance, and chest radiograph appearance [31]. A score of greater than 3 defined severe respiratory failure. Survival without disability was significantly higher in the patients referred to an ECMO center (63% vs. 47%) [28]. However, limitations of the study in evaluating the actual efficacy of ECMO for severe ARDS included the lack of a homogenous ventilation strategy in the control group, and a high percentage of patients that were referred to the ECMO center but never placed on ECMO (25%).

The ECMO to rescue Lung Injury in severe ARDS (EOLIA) trial studied 249 patients with severe ARDS who received either early venovenous (VV) ECMO or conventional LTTV with late ECMO as a rescue modality [29]. Severe ARDS was defined as a $PaO_2:FiO_2$ < 50 mm Hg for >3 h or $PaO_2:FiO_2$ < 80 mm Hg for >6 h. The group receiving early ECMO was placed as soon as criteria for severe ARDS were met. The data safety and monitoring board overseeing the study stopped the trial early when interim results were largely in favor of ECMO [32]. However, in the final analysis the primary outcome of 60-day mortality, which remained in favor of ECMO, was not statistically significant (46% vs. 35%) [29]. Survival was also much higher in those who received ECMO within 2 days after onset of ARDS vs. those who received it later within about 6 days after onset (65% vs. 43%). Early cessation of the trial along with a high percentage of patients that crossed over from conventional LTTV to ECMO as a rescue modality may have biased the results away from benefits associated with early ECMO use.

During the H1N1 influenza pandemic of 2009, a study of 75 patients with severe ARDS was conducted in a matched pair design [30]. It found that transfer of patients to an ECMO center improved survival considerably (76.3% vs. 47.5%). 85% of transferred patients were placed on ECMO during the study.

One of the major limitations to conducting well controlled studies in this niche is the relative paucity in numbers of severe ARDS patients necessitating the coordination of large multicenter networks amongst relatively few centers with ample ECMO experience. This comes at great expense of time and resources and, as in the case of the EOLIA trial, risks underpowering of the study when looking at important differences in outcomes. Several meta-analyses have attempted to overcome these limitations. One of these reviewed two randomized trials and three observational studies, finding that 60-day survival was higher in severe ARDS patients who received VV ECMO (66% vs. 53%; RR 0.73, 95% CI 0.58–0.92) [33]. Using a Bayesian random-effects network metanalysis, another study reviewed 25 randomized clinical trials ranking the relative effectiveness of 9 different interventions (including ECMO) in moderate to severe ARDS patients undergoing lung protective ventilation [23]. The two interventions with the highest-ranking probabilities of significantly lowering 28-day mortality compared with LTVV alone were prone positioning (PP) and VV ECMO (PP: RR 0.69, 95% CI 0.48–0.99; VV ECMO: RR 0.60, 95% CI 0.38–0.93). Finally, a meta-analysis that looked at pooled data from both the CESAR and EOLIA trials found a 90-day reduced mortality in patients who received ECMO (RR 0.75, 95% CI 0.6–0.94) [34].

The SARS-CoV-2 pandemic spanning the last few years has dramatically increased experience across critical care centers around the world in managing patients with severe ARDS, including in the use of ECMO for the most severe cases. Initial observations by some experts suggested COVID ARDS was much different in its need for lung protective strategies compared to non-COVID-related disease [35]. However, subsequent detailed analyses revealed a similar distribution of severity, lung compliances, recruitment thresholds, and response to lung protective measures, leading expert consensus back towards recommending the use of well-established lung protective strategies in COVID ARDS [35].

Due to a temporary increase in large numbers of patients with very severe forms of ARDS worldwide, experience with the use of ECMO in ARDS has grown during the pandemic. While the opportunity for controlled studies has been limited, much of this experience has been reported via observational series and retrospective studies.

A retrospective cohort study conducted in Wuhan, China, on critically ill COVID-19 patients between January 2020 and March 2020 concluded that those who received ECMO had significantly lower in-hospital mortality rates compared to those who received conventional therapy (58.8% vs. 93.5%, $P = 0.001$) [36]. Further analysis of the cause of death between these two groups revealed that zero of the patients in the ECMO group died from ARDS (0 vs. 51.6%, $P = 0.000$). When death occurred in the ECMO group it was more likely to be related to sepsis (17.6% vs. 0, $P = 0.025$). No differences were observed between the two groups for all other causes of death. The most common complication noted in the ECMO group was bleeding (84% of patients in ECMO group) [36].

Blazoski et al. noted in their literature review how poor the overall mortality of COVID-ARDS was compared to influenza-ARDS [37]. For instance, those admitted to the ICU with COVID have a 3.7 times higher risk of death than those who are admitted for influenza. Similar outcomes were found in Veteran's Affairs Hospitals, in which the risk of death was noted to be 5 times higher in those admitted for COVID than for influenza [37]. To see how ECMO affected these statistics, Blazoski et al. looked at the outcomes of ECMO in influenza vs. COVID patients during the first wave of the COVID-19 pandemic. Patients with ARDS secondary to either influenza or COVID-19 that were placed on ECMO between August 1, 2010 through September 15, 2020 were compared in this retrospective study. Twenty-eight COVID patients and 17 influenza patients were included in this study with the survival rates being overall better in the influenza group compared to the COVID group (94% vs. 68%, respectively ($P = 0.04$) [37]. Further analysis of 30-day survival following VV ECMO decannulation also favored the influenza group compared to the COVID group, being 76% vs. 54% respectively. However, this finding was not statistically significant ($P = 0.13$). This study found that COVID patients tended to spend more time on ECMO support (21 days vs. 12 days, $P = 0.25$) and had higher rates of new infection (50% vs. 18%, $P = 0.03$) and bacterial pneumonia (36% vs. 8%, $P = 0.24$) when compared to their influenza counterparts [37]. COVID patients in this study were more likely to have received immunomodulatory therapy prior to ECMO initiation as part of their treatment, which may have played a role in their higher infection risk.

Jäckel et al. conducted an analysis looking at the use of VV ECMO in COVID-19 ARDS as compared to influenza related ARDS in a retrospective study of patients managed between October 2010 and June 2020 [38]. At 30 days following ECMO cannulation, 13.35% of COVID-19 ARDS patients vs. 44.7% with influenza were discharged alive from their ICU ($P = 0.03$). COVID-19 patients were also more likely to have fewer VV ECMO free days and longer ICU treatment duration than their influenza counterparts. 30-day mortality was noted to be higher in the COVID-19 group but wasn't found to be statistically significant. This may have been secondary to a smaller number of cases in the COVID group compared to the influenza group (15 vs. 47) [38].

Given the high cost in labor and other resources that are associated with ECMO support, prediction models of survival on ECMO have long been sought, and experience during the pandemic expanded knowledge specifically for severe ARDS patients. Zayat et al. conducted a single-center, retrospective observational study examining all severe COVID-ARDS patients who received ECMO support between March 1, 2020 to April 20, 2020 [39]. A total of 83 pre-ECMO variables including biomarkers, risk scores, and demographics were evaluated for predictiveness of survival. Procalcitonin, IL-6 and NT-proBNP were all remarkably higher in non-survivors versus survivors. Data also validated the Respiratory Extracorporeal Membrane Oxygenation (RESP) Score [40] as a viable survival prediction tool for patients with severe COVID ARDS who undergo ECMO support.

Optimal timing of ECMO initiation for severe ARDS is also a matter of ongoing debate, with some experts favoring early institution when it appears that lung protective strategies will not be viable on the basis of severe acidosis and/or hypoxemia, while others favor its institution only after all other lung protective strategies have been attempted. Two studies conducted during the pandemic have contributed to this debate.

A cohort research study conducted by Giraud et al. included COVID-19 ARDS patients admitted to the Geneva University Hospital ICU between March 14 and May 31, 2020, who were supported on VV ECMO [41]. Amongst the 10 patients studied, mean durations of mechanical ventilation and ECMO were 7 ± 3 days and 19 ± 11 days, respectively. Six patients died in the cohort, leaving the study mortality at 60%. This study highlighted that survivors had a significantly shorter duration on mechanical ventilation prior to ECMO initiation compared to non-survivors (91 ± 58 h vs. 208 ± 34 h, $P = 0.01$) as well as a shorter amount of time on

Study	Characteristics	Main Findings	Citation
CESAR	RCT of Severe ARDS patient randomized to ECMO or conventional therapy	Survival without disability higher in ECMO group (63% vs. 47%)	doi: 10.1186/1472-6963-6-163
EOLIA	RCT of Severe ARDS patients randomized to early ECMO vs. conventional LTVV with potential for late ECMO initiation	Survival higher in ECMO group who were initiated 2 days after onset of ARDS vs. those who were initiated within 6 days after diagnosis (65% vs. 43%)	doi:10.1056/NEJMoa1800385
Li et al.	Retrospective study of COVID-19 patients who received VV ECMO	COVID-19 patients who received ECMO had better mortality rates than those who received conventional therapy -COVID-19 patients who received ECMO did not die from ARDS but rather from sepsis/infection	doi: 10.1111/jocs.15833
Blazoski et al.	Retrospective study to evaluate outcomes of ECMO in influenza ARDS vs. COVID ARDS	Influenza ARDS had better survival rates with ECMO than COVID-19 ARDS treated with ECMO	doi: 10.1111/jocs.15888
Jackel et al.	Retrospective study evaluating difference in outcomes of influenza ARDS on ECMO vs. COVID-19 ARDS on ECMO	Longer VV ECMO duration and ICU duration noted in COVID-19 ARDS group	doi: 10.1111/aor.13865
Zayat et al.	Retrospective observational study of COVID-19 patients to determine predictors of survival	Elevated procalcitonin, IL-6 and NT-proBNP associated with mortality -High RESP score associated with greater chance of survival	doi: 10.1111/aor.13873
Giraud et al.	Observational and retrospective cohort study evaluating how timing of ECMO initiation influences outcomes	It is likely futile to initiate ECMO in severe COVID-19 ARDS patients who have been on mechanical ventilation for 7 days or more -patients with this profile in their study ultimately died	doi: 10.14814/phy2.14715
Kurihara et al.	Retrospective cohort study of -COVID-19 vs. non-COVID-19 ARDS and how to determine optimal timing of support initiation	100% of COVID-19 patients initiated on ECMO after 7 days died -non-COVID-19 ARDS have better odds at survival even if initiation of ECMO is delayed after 7 days (30.7% mortality)	doi: 10.1111/aor.14090

Presented in order as they appear in chapter.

Table 1.
Summary of studies.

ECMO (246 ± 102 days vs. 588 ± 294 days, $P = 0.038$) and in the ICU (17 ± 6 days vs. 32 ± 12 days, $P = 0.016$). Overall, this meant that those who received longer than 7 days on mechanical ventilation prior to initiation of ECMO in their study ultimately died. The study found no other pre-ECMO variable that was statistically significant in predicting survival. The investigators concluded that ECMO is a viable option for refractory hypoxemia in COVID-19 patients with ARDS, but that it should be considered early in their clinical course, as late initiation of ECMO therapy (beyond 7 days of mechanical ventilation) is likely futile [41].

The other retrospective cohort study contributing to the debate around timing was conducted by Kurihara et al. [42]. They similarly reported that COVID-19 ARDS patients who received more than 7 days of mechanical ventilation prior to VV-ECMO initiation had a very high mortality rate. In this study mortality was 100% when ECMO initiation was delayed beyond 7 days of mechanical ventilation. The COVID-19 ARDS patients who received 7 days or less of mechanical ventilation had a 63.1% mortality rate compared to 30.7% in the non-COVID-19 ARDS group. The investigators were unable to determine why the 7-day cut off was so significant. Since COVID-19 patients typically experience multiple episodes of proning, they decided to evaluate if the increased number of proning episodes in COVID-19 patients prior to VV ECMO cannulation affected post-ECMO mortality. They did not find a specific number of proning episodes that predicted mortality post-ECMO in the COVID-19 cohort.

4. Conclusion

Taken altogether, the preponderance of research in the field has clearly demonstrated an exquisite sensitivity of the ARDS lung to stretch-mediated injury with strong signals for increased mortality when lung protective strategies are abandoned. It follows that in select cases of extremely severe ARDS, a role for extracorporeal support exists in which the injured lung is allowed to rest and recover. Although more work needs to be done, this hypothesis is supported by the current cache of clinical research observations including those derived from experiences during the COVID-19 pandemic (**Table 1**). In response to this data, current guidelines established by the international Extracorporeal Life Support Organization (ELSO) suggest consideration of ECMO in patients with severe ARDS and refractory hypoxemia ($PaO_2/FiO_2 < 80$ mm Hg), or severe hypercapnic acidosis (pH < 7.25 with a $PaCO_2 \geq 60$ mm Hg) after optimal conventional management including a trial of prone positioning (in the absence of contraindications) [43]. Since increased duration of mechanical ventilation prior to the institution of ECMO is associated with worsened mortality, it is also recommended that optimal medical management be rapidly and maximally implemented, and transition to ECMO performed without delay when indicated. The only absolute contraindication to the use of ECMO in severe ARDS is anticipated nonrecovery without a feasible plan for decannulation or possibility of bridge to transplantation [43].

As advancements in ECMO device technology and implementation experience continue to reduce complication rates, it is anticipated that future research will be sufficiently powered to definitively refine optimal patient selection and timing of ECMO implementation in severe ARDS. Advancements in single site cannulation methods, device portability, and experience managing patients on VV ECMO without mechanical ventilation have allowed inroads to be made with regards to safe mobility-promoting therapy during extended ECMO support [44], which is independently associated with improved outcomes during critical illness [45]. It is hoped that these efforts will culminate in continued reductions in the high mortality rates associated with this otherwise devastating condition.

Acknowledgements

This work was supported by NIH 1 K08 HL140222-01A1 to SS.

Author details

Ashley K. Binder and Sunit Singla*
Division of Pulmonary, Critical Care, Sleep, and Allergy Medicine, Department of Medicine, University of Illinois, Chicago, IL, USA

*Address all correspondence to: ssingl6@uic.edu

References

[1] Ranieri VM et al. Acute respiratory distress syndrome: The Berlin definition. JAMA. 2012;**307**(23):2526-2533

[2] Gattinoni L et al. Regional effects and mechanism of positive end-expiratory pressure in early adult respiratory distress syndrome. JAMA. 1993;**269**(16):2122-2127

[3] Pelosi P et al. Vertical gradient of regional lung inflation in adult respiratory distress syndrome. American Journal of Respiratory and Critical Care Medicine. 1994;**149**(1):8-13

[4] Brower RG, et al. Ventilation with lower tidal volumes as compared with traditional tidal volumes for acute lung injury and the acute respiratory distress syndrome. New England Journal of Medicine. 2000;**342**(18):1301-1308

[5] Gattinoni L et al. The "baby lung" became an adult. Intensive Care Medicine. 2016;**42**(5):663-673

[6] Needham DM et al. Lung protective mechanical ventilation and two year survival in patients with acute lung injury: Prospective cohort study. British Medical Journal. 2012;**344**:e2124

[7] Needham DM et al. Timing of low tidal volume ventilation and intensive care unit mortality in acute respiratory distress syndrome. A prospective cohort study. American Journal of Respiratory and Critical Care Medicine. 2015;**191**(2):177-185

[8] Petrucci N, De Feo C. Lung protective ventilation strategy for the acute respiratory distress syndrome. The Cochrane Database of Systematic Reviews. 2013;**2013**(2):Cd003844

[9] Kellner M et al. ROS Signaling in the pathogenesis of acute lung injury (ALI) and acute respiratory distress syndrome (ARDS). Advances in Experimental Medicine and Biology. 2017;**967**:105-137

[10] Investigators W.G.f.t.A.R.f.A.R.D.S.T. Effect of lung recruitment and titrated positive end-expiratory pressure (PEEP) vs low PEEP on mortality in patients with acute respiratory distress syndrome: A randomized clinical trial. JAMA. 2017;**318**(14):1335-1345

[11] Gattinoni L et al. What has computed tomography taught us about the acute respiratory distress syndrome? American Journal of Respiratory and Critical Care Medicine. 2001;**164**(9):1701-1711

[12] Gattinoni L et al. Lung recruitment in patients with the acute respiratory distress syndrome. The New England Journal of Medicine. 2006;**354**(17):1775-1786

[13] Grasso S et al. Effects of recruiting maneuvers in patients with acute respiratory distress syndrome ventilated with protective ventilatory strategy. Anesthesiology. 2002;**96**(4):795-802

[14] Kallet RH. A comprehensive review of prone position in ARDS. Respiratory Care. 2015;**60**(11):1660-1687

[15] Galiatsou E et al. Prone position augments recruitment and prevents alveolar overinflation in acute lung injury. American Journal of Respiratory and Critical Care Medicine. 2006;**174**(2):187-197

[16] Guérin C et al. Prone positioning in severe acute respiratory distress syndrome. New England Journal of Medicine. 2013;**368**(23):2159-2168

[17] Bloomfield R, Noble DW, Sudlow A. Prone position for acute respiratory

failure in adults. The Cochrane Database of Systematic Reviews. 2015;**2015**(11):Cd008095

[18] Sud S et al. Prone ventilation reduces mortality in patients with acute respiratory failure and severe hypoxemia: Systematic review and meta-analysis. Intensive Care Medicine. 2010;**36**(4):585-599

[19] Hu SL et al. The effect of prone positioning on mortality in patients with acute respiratory distress syndrome: A meta-analysis of randomized controlled trials. Critical Care. 2014;**18**(3):R109

[20] Park SY et al. The efficacy and safety of prone positioning in adults patients with acute respiratory distress syndrome: A meta-analysis of randomized controlled trials. Journal of Thoracic Disease. 2015;**7**(3):356-367

[21] Munshi L et al. Prone position for acute respiratory distress syndrome. a systematic review and meta-analysis. Annals of the American Thoracic Society. 2017;**14**(Supplement_4):S280-S288

[22] Sud S et al. Comparative effectiveness of protective ventilation strategies for moderate and severe acute respiratory distress syndrome. A network Meta-analysis. American Journal of Respiratory and Critical Care Medicine. 2021;**203**(11):1366-1377

[23] Aoyama H et al. Assessment of therapeutic interventions and lung protective ventilation in patients with moderate to severe acute respiratory distress syndrome: A systematic review and network Meta-analysis. JAMA Network Open. 2019;**2**(7):e198116

[24] Yoshida T et al. Spontaneous effort causes occult pendelluft during mechanical ventilation. American Journal of Respiratory and Critical Care Medicine. 2013;**188**(12):1420-1427

[25] Papazian L et al. Neuromuscular blockers in early acute respiratory distress syndrome. New England Journal of Medicine. 2010;**363**(12):1107-1116

[26] Moss M, etal. Early neuromuscular blockade in the acute respiratory distress syndrome. New England Journal of Medicine. 2019;**380**(21):1997-2008

[27] Force T.A.D.T. Acute respiratory distress syndrome: The Berlin definition. JAMA. 2012;**307**(23):2526-2533

[28] Peek GJ et al. Efficacy and economic assessment of conventional ventilatory support versus extracorporeal membrane oxygenation for severe adult respiratory failure (CESAR): A multicentre randomised controlled trial. The Lancet. 2009;**374**(9698):1351-1363

[29] Combes A et al. Extracorporeal membrane oxygenation for severe acute respiratory distress syndrome. The New England Journal of Medicine. 2018;**378**(21):1965-1975

[30] Noah MA et al. Referral to an extracorporeal membrane oxygenation center and mortality among patients with severe 2009 influenza A(H1N1). JAMA. 2011;**306**(15):1659-1668

[31] Murray JF et al. An expanded definition of the adult respiratory distress syndrome. The American Review of Respiratory Disease. 1988;**138**(3): 720-723

[32] Harrington D, Drazen JM. Learning from a trial stopped by a data and safety monitoring board. The New England Journal of Medicine. 2018;**378**(21):2031-2032

[33] Munshi L et al. Venovenous extracorporeal membrane oxygenation for acute respiratory distress syndrome: A systematic review and meta-analysis.

The Lancet Respiratory Medicine. 2019;7(2):163-172

[34] Combes A et al. ECMO for severe ARDS: Systematic review and individual patient data meta-analysis. Intensive Care Medicine. 2020;**46**(11):2048-2057

[35] Fan E et al. COVID-19-associated acute respiratory distress syndrome: Is a different approach to management warranted? The Lancet Respiratory Medicine. 2020;**8**(8):816-821

[36] Li S et al. Extracorporeal membrane oxygenation (ECMO) for critically ill patients with coronavirus disease 2019 (COVID-19): A retrospective cohort study. Journal of Cardiac Surgery. 2021;**36**(10):3554-3560

[37] Blazoski CM et al. Outcomes of extracorporeal membrane oxygenation in influenza versus COVID-19 during the first wave of COVID-19. Journal of Cardiac Surgery. 2021;**36**(10):3740-3746

[38] Jäckel M et al. Outcome of acute respiratory distress syndrome requiring extracorporeal membrane oxygenation in Covid-19 or influenza: A single-center registry study. Artificial Organs. 2021;**45**(6):593-601

[39] Zayat R et al. Role of extracorporeal membrane oxygenation in critically ill COVID-19 patients and predictors of mortality. Artificial Organs. 2021;**45**(6):E158-E170

[40] Schmidt M et al. Predicting survival after extracorporeal membrane oxygenation for severe acute respiratory failure. The respiratory extracorporeal membrane oxygenation survival prediction (RESP) score. American Journal of Respiratory and Critical Care Medicine. 2014;**189**(11):1374-1382

[41] Giraud R et al. Timing of VV-ECMO therapy implementation influences prognosis of COVID-19 patients. Physiological Reports. 2021;**9**(3):e14715

[42] Kurihara C et al. Outcomes after extracorporeal membrane oxygenation support in COVID-19 and non-COVID-19 patients. Artificial Organs. 2022;**46**(4):688-696

[43] Tonna JE et al. Management of adult patients supported with venovenous extracorporeal membrane oxygenation (VV ECMO): Guideline from the extracorporeal life support organization (ELSO). ASAIO Journal. 2021;**67**(6):601-610

[44] Abrams D et al. Early mobilization during extracorporeal membrane oxygenation for cardiopulmonary failure in adults: Factors associated with intensity of treatment. Annals of the American Thoracic Society. 2022;**19**(1):90-98

[45] Cameron S et al. Early mobilization in the critical care unit: A review of adult and pediatric literature. Journal of Critical Care. 2015;**30**(4):664-672

Chapter 10

The Role of VV-ECMO in Severe COVID-19 ARDS

Cathal MacDonncha, Rachel Jooste, John Laffey and Ciara Hanley

Abstract

Although an established practice in potentially reversible severe respiratory failure, extracorporeal membrane oxygenation (ECMO) support remains controversial. Over the last 50 years, only 4 large scale randomised controlled trials relating to ECMO have been conducted in patients with ARDS. A meta-analysis of only 2 studies has demonstrated survival benefit in those supported with ECMO compared to optimal conventional therapy. With the advent of the COVID pandemic, ECMO utilisation increased, the guidelines evolved, and an unprecedented number of patients were referred for and managed with ECMO support. Approximately 15,000 patients have been supported to date, predominantly using veno-venous ECMO, with an overall in-hospital 90-day mortality of 47%. Although published data reported an increase in ECMO mortality to nearly 60% as the pandemic progressed, this was likely multifactorial, as subsequent data has demonstrated more promising mortality results. This highlights the unique challenges pertaining to patient selection and implementation of this finite support amid an evolving pandemic with many unknowns. Judicious and ethical patient selection is essential to ensure use for the greatest benefit. In this chapter we will outline the unique pathophysiology and clinical features of COVID-ARDS, indications for ECMO referral and patient selection, and implementation during the COVID-19 pandemic.

Keywords: COVID-19, ARDS, VV ECMO, COVID-19 pathophysiology, hypoxaemia

1. Introduction

With the outbreak of COVID, extracorporeal membrane oxygen support (ECMO) utilisation exponentially increased, and the guidelines on ECMO referral, selection, and patient management rapidly evolved to cope with the unprecedented scale of the pandemic [1]. To date, an unparalleled number of patients have been referred for and managed with ECMO. According to the Extracorporeal Life Support Organisation (ELSO) COVID-19 ECMO registry, approximately 15,000 patients have been supported so far, predominantly using veno-venous ECMO (VV ECMO), with an overall in-hospital 90-day mortality of 47% [2]. Although the pandemic led to an upscale in ECMO use, ECMO mortality actually increased to nearly 60% as the pandemic progressed over 2020 [3]. However, this increase is likely a function of multiple interconnected factors as more recent mortality data has been more optimistic with an estimated survival probability of 87% on Day 7 ECMO and 78% at 90-days, compared with 83% and 64% respectively in the conventional management group [4]. The type of variant, patient demographic and comorbidity, a more severe COVID-ARDS phenotype and lack of reversibility, increased and/ or more resistant co-infections (some of which are possibly associated with steroids and novel COVID-19 therapies), and treatment in a low vs. high volume ECMO centre may have contributed to this mortality variance. The inconsistency in patient outcomes highlights the unique challenges pertaining to judicious and ethical patient selection, and appropriate application of this expensive and finite mode of support amid an evolving pandemic with many unknowns in order to ensure its use for the greatest benefit.

2. Background

2.1 An overview of COVID-19 pathophysiology

Since its isolation in December 2019 in Wuhan China, the novel severe acute respiratory syndrome coronavirus-2 (SARS-CoV-2), and its resultant syndrome COVID-19, have affected nearly 567 million people across the globe, with a death toll of over 6 million according to the latest data from the World Health Organisation [5]. Its clinical presentation has been variable, ranging from asymptomatic “happy hypoxaemia”, to one of refractory severe acute respiratory failure in the intensive care unit requiring potentially lifesaving extracorporeal support. Approximately 20% of patients with COVID-19 develop severe COVID pneumonitis, which is similar to conventional acute respiratory distress syndrome (ARDS) as defined by the Berlin criteria [6, 7].

Severe COVID-19 is the consequence of a virally triggered cytokine storm, resulting in initial endothelial inflammation and hypercoagulopathy, rapidly followed by pulmonary oedema, progressive lung parenchymal consolidation, diffuse alveolar damage, and pulmonary fibrosis. The interaction between the SARS-CoV-2 spike proteins and the angiotensin converting enzyme-2 (ACE2) receptor present on type 2 pneumocytes via receptor-mediated endocytosis, has been postulated as the fundamental mechanism driving this cytokine response [8]. Although patients generally present with isolated respiratory failure, progression to multiorgan failure may be rapid. COVID-related multiorgan failure and secondary infection related multiorgan failure are the leading causes of mortality, accounting for 37% and 26% of deaths respectively [9]. A hypercoagulable state is particularly common, and is reflected by increased fibrinogen and D-dimer levels in almost all patients, with a concomitant increased incidence of both venous and arterial thrombosis, pulmonary thromboembolism, and associated increased mortality [10]. Post-mortem studies have demonstrated that the histological hallmark of COVID ARDS is diffuse alveolar infiltration with varying degrees of pulmonary vascular thrombosis [11–13].

2.2 Hypoxaemia and respiratory system compliance

Although there is progressive hypoxaemia and dyspnoea, the hypoxaemia in COVID-19 is often more severe than that expected from the anatomical shunt alone. In fact, despite a PaO2/FiO2 ratio < 200 mmHg (26.7 kPa) in moderate-to-severe disease, approximately 40–50% of patients have preserved respiratory system compliance (CRS), with peripherally distributed ground glass opacification and minimal parenchymal consolidation, which is in stark contrast to the majority of non-COVID ARDS [14]. There is a small subgroup of classic ARDS that may have high compliance [15]. The underlying mechanisms for the disproportionate hypoxaemia are multifactorial, determined by a temporal and spatial heterogeneous mismatch of pulmonary ventilation and perfusion, a loss of hypoxic pulmonary vasoconstriction, and dysregulated pulmonary blood flow, mainly associated with immunothrombosis, endothelial inflammation and neovascularisation [16–18].

COVID-19 patients tend to have preserved CRS despite significant pulmonary fibrosis, pulmonary infiltration, pulmonary vascular micro and/ or macro thrombosis and resulting hypoxaemic respiratory failure. A range of clinical phenotypes may exist. Maiolo et al. proposed 3 distinct groups. Firstly, a high elastance-poor compliance group ("H-type") with a CRS < 40 ml/cm H_2O, increased right-to-left shunt, increased lung weight, and potentially more recruitable lung. This group accounts for 20–30% of COVID ARDS patients in critical care [19]. The second group is "Intermediate CRS", defined as a compliance of 40–50 ml/cm H_2O, and finally a reduced elastance group ("L-type") characterised by preserved/ high compliance (CRS >50 ml/cm H_2O), low ventilation-perfusion ratio, low lung weight, and minimal recruitable lung. Camporota et al. have proposed that the earlier phase of COVID ARDS is characterised by a high compliance phenotype, with a transition to a poorer compliance state as the disease progresses [20]. However, further data has questioned the phenotype concept. Several single centre observational studies, including the recent COVADIS study, have demonstrated that the mean CRS is actually rather poor, c. 30–40 mL/cm H_2O. The COVADIS results demonstrated a unimodal distribution of CRS around a mean value of 37 ml/ cm H_2O, similar to that observed in non-COVID-19 ARDS. CRS decreased from day 1 to day 14, and interestingly patients with higher CRS did not demonstrate faster weaning of mechanical ventilation or increased survival in multivariate analyses [21]. Ferrando et al. demonstrated a similar mean CRS distribution of 35 ml/cm H_2O (IQR: 27–45). However, their findings were likely limited by a high proportion of incomplete data [22]. Factors that may partly explain some of the variability in compliance data may be the time since disease onset and time from disease onset to intubation. Early in the pandemic, intubation tended to occur based on hypoxaemia alone. However, as the pandemic progressed, intubation was often deferred until more clinical disease progression occurred at which point compliance would have been poor, and of a more typical ARDS nature. Mortality in COVID-ARDS does however correlate with poorer compliance (CRS < 48 ml/cm H_2O) and increased driving pressure, independent of tidal volume per kilogramme based on ideal body weight, and even with tidal volumes above the accepted 6–8 ml/kg threshold [23]. Notably, patients with COVID ARDS who have a reduced CRS together with increased D-dimer concentrations have a worse survival prognosis [14].

2.3 Pulmonary hypertension

Pulmonary hypertension leading to acute right ventricular (RV) dysfunction +/− failure may occur in COVID ARDS and is associated with a significantly increased mortality (48.5% versus 24.7% in patients with and without RV dysfunction respectively; 56.3% versus 30.6% in patients with or without RV dilatation). Mortality is high even in patients with pulmonary hypertension (PH) without RV strain (52.9% versus 14.8%) [24]. The underlying mechanism is primarily an increase in RV afterload due to increased pulmonary vascular resistance (PVR). Multiple factors in COVID ARDS contribute to PH, elevated PVR, increased RV afterload and, eventually, RV failure. These include hypoxaemia, hypercapnia, acidosis, hypoxic pulmonary vasoconstriction, endothelial inflammation, pulmonary vascular thrombosis, and vascular remodelling. RV dilatation increases the RV distending pressure, thereby increasing the pressure gradient for subendocardial myocardial perfusion, resulting in impaired RV contractility. Pressure volume overload consequently impairs left ventricular function and cardiac output. Although possibly more severe in COVID-19 ARDS, RV dysfunction can be alleviated by improving gas exchange with VV ECMO [25].

2.4 Management principles in severe COVID-19

The management of severe COVID-ARDS is multimodal, and the intensity of support required depends on the phenotype and severity of the disease at presentation. Potentially reversible severe COVID pneumonitis that is refractory to protective lung ventilation, ventilatory adjuncts i.e., prone positioning, inhaled pulmonary vasodilators, neuromuscular blockade etc., and also to targeted pharmacological therapy i.e., steroids, immunotherapy, and antimicrobial agents may require extracorporeal membrane support oxygenation as a bridge to recovery or in exceptional cases, lung transplantation [26]. Venovenous (VV) ECMO support is the modality of choice in 95.9% of cases, as demonstrated in a systematic review and meta-analysis of 18,211 COVID-19 patients by Ling et al. [27] ECMO may also represent an efficient support in cases of severe cardiogenic/septic shock refractory to maximal therapy in these patients. However, venoarterial (VA) ECMO, conversion to VA ECMO from VV ECMO, or use of hybrid ECMO circuits are rare in COVID-19, accounting for <5% of all cases [27]. It is also important to consider that patients with other potential indications for ECMO support, such as massive pulmonary embolism, myocarditis or acute myocardial infarction, may also be COVID-19 positive [28]. Although seen as an established therapy in potentially reversible severe respiratory failure, ECMO remains controversial. Over the last 50 years, only 4 large scale randomised controlled trials have been conducted in patients with non-COVID-ARDS [29–32]. Overall, these studies have not demonstrated superiority of ECMO over maximal conventional support i.e., protective lung ventilation, prone positioning etc. However, a meta-analysis of the CESAR and EOLIA studies demonstrated a 90-day mortality benefit in the ECMO group (36% vs. 48%; relative risk, 0.75, 95% confidence interval 0.6–0.94; $p = 0.013$), in addition to more ventilator free days and days out of ICU [33].

3. Referral, patient selection, and ethics

ECMO is a complex and resource intensive intervention. Its use is mostly restricted to specialist centres globally. Disease severity, reversibility and patient reserve are important aspects when considering suitability for ECMO. Selection of patients who will ultimately benefit most is crucial to avoid suffering and prolonged futile ICU admission, in addition to appropriate allocation of an expensive, finite, and labour-intensive resource.

ECMO played a crucial role in previous respiratory viral outbreaks, such as the Middle East Respiratory Syndrome coronavirus (MERS-CoV2) in 2012, and the influenza A virus subtype hemagglutinin 1 neuraminidase 1 in 2009 (H1N1), with acceptable survival rates ranging from 65% to 77% [34]. However, it was clear from the start of the COVID-19, that this global outbreak would place an even greater strain on healthcare systems worldwide in comparison with its predecessors. Early in the pandemic, definitive data to guide clinical decision making for patient selection in severe COVID-19 was lacking, and established protocols for the initiation of VV ECMO in COVID-19 were therefore largely based on 2 randomised controlled trials of ECMO for non-COVID ARDS [29, 30]. As pandemic phases evolved, ELSO adapted its guideline recommendations in this regard [1]. The 2020 ELSO guidelines, the 2021 ELSO update, and guidelines from other international bodies recommended that VV ECMO should be considered in all patients with COVID-19 and severe refractory hypoxaemia despite optimal conventional therapy [1, 35–38].

Providing complex, finite, and resource intensive therapies such as ECMO during a pandemic has unique challenges [39]. During COVID, referral and selection criteria for VV ECMO had to be redefined during essential resource planning and allocation in order to ethically deploy finite resources. A better understanding of the disease process developed as the pandemic progressed, allowing dynamic modification of these criteria. As a result, regional ECMO services developed individualised approaches to patient selection with a unified aim to ensure that ECMO is offered to those patients who are more likely to reap the most benefit [34, 40, 41]. There is however, some heterogeneity in published selection criteria based on regional variations in demographics, pandemic phase, and resource availability [34, 41].

3.1 Referral criteria

Referral for ECMO (**Table 1**) should be considered in any COVID-19 patient with potentially reversible acute hypoxaemic respiratory failure, defined as a PaO2/FiO2 ratio < 80 mm Hg, refractory to maximal conventional therapy as per the ELSO recommended algorithm i.e. treatment of underlying cause, protective lung ventilation, diuresis; followed by prone positioning, increased PEEP, use of neuromuscular blockade, and inhaled pulmonary vasodilators +/− recruitment manoeuvres [1]. Severity of hypoxemia in COVID-19 respiratory failure is characterised by the partial pressure of arterial oxygen to fraction of inspired oxygen (PaO2/FiO2) ratio using thresholds recommended in the EOLIA trial [30]. Early referral is particularly important for patients deteriorating in non-ECMO centres. Referral should be made as early as possible in advance of further deterioration to facilitate timely retrieval and transfer to the designated ECMO centre. ECMO initiation should not be delayed due to resource constraints; delays in initiation are associated with increased mortality in both COVID and non-COVID ARDS [1, 42, 43]. There is no consensus on absolute contraindications for referral in COVID ARDS, except in cases of end-stage respiratory failure unsuitable for lung transplantation, and also when critical care system capacity is at crisis point. The optimal timing of ECMO initiation in relation to intubation remains debatable. In non-COVID ARDS, a duration of mechanical ventilation of 7 days or longer is considered to increase the likelihood of irreversibility [29, 33]. Contrary to this, as discussed in detail below, there is emerging evidence that this has minimal impact on mortality in COVID-19 patients supported with ECMO. However, it is still reasonable to assume based on the available evidence, that earlier initiation is associated with improved survival [34, 40, 41, 44]. Of note, high intensity and prolonged non-invasive ventilation (NIV) in an attempt to avoid intubation during the second wave resulted in delayed initiation of evidenced based lung protective ventilation with an increased incidence of barotrauma. Referral criteria were redefined by some ECMO experts to consider days of high intensity continuous positive airway

1. Refractory severe hypoxaemia PaO2/FiO2 ratio < 80 mmHg for >6 hours *OR* PaO2/FiO2 ratio < 50 mmHg for >3 hours
+/− pH < 7.25
+/− PaCO2 > 60 mmHg for >6 hours
2. Uncompensated refractory severe hypercapnia, with or without severe hypoxaemia (PaO2/FiO2 < 150 mmHg)
*Respiratory rate increased to 35 *Plateau pressure < 32cmH20
3. Lung Injury Score ≥ 3
PLUS
4. Failure of optimal protective lung ventilation and adjunctive therapy
5. Absence of contraindications to extracorporeal support
6. Thorough discussion with a national ECMO centre
Adapted from Badulak et al. [1], Dalia et al. [34], Camporota et al. [41].

Table 1.
Referral criteria for VV ECMO in severe refractory COVID-19.

pressure (CPAP) or non-invasive ventilation (NIV) as days of mechanical ventilation in an attempt to encourage early referral [41].

3.2 Patient selection

Given the required judicious approach to patient selection during a pandemic with finite resources, how do we determine who will benefit most? Risk factors for poor survival have been identified and are further discussed in the section on mortality and morbidity. Overall, increasing age, ECMO centre experience and pre-existing concomitant disease are substantial factors congruent worldwide. These factors, in addition to premorbid functional capacity, must be considered during the process of referral and when deciding to initiate ECMO, in order to determine a realistic survival and rehabilitation potential, and also expected quality of life after ECMO. For patients with challenging considerations or potential relative contraindications (**Table 2**), it would be reasonable to suggest that at least two ECMO centres should agree that it is appropriate to proceed to ECMO in these cases.

3.3 Ethics and ECMO in a pandemic

Although there has been intense debate regarding ethical allocation of critical care resources during the COVID-19 pandemic, there has been a paucity of professional guidance specifically relating to ethics and ECMO allocation, with the notable exception of a general ethical guidance document published by ELSO in May 2020 [45]. An international survey of ECMO practitioners (primarily from the ECMOCard group) during the early stages of the pandemic has shed some light on the current ethical climate. Probability of survival if treated, pre-existing disability, functional status, and patient age were the most cited discriminating factors in decision making around maximising patient survival benefit when considering suitability for

	Recommended	Consider in individual cases**	Not indicated
Age (years)	<65	65–69	No definitive consensus But >70 is associated with much higher mortality
Comorbidity	No significant comorbidity	Immunosuppression (within 6 months prior)	BMI > 35
		Recent neurosurgical procedure	Refusal of blood products or anticoagulation
		Renal failure	Documented end-stage chronic organ failure (e.g., COPD, cirrhosis); not for device therapy or transplant
			Severe acute neurological injury with poor prognosis for recovery
			Active malignancy
			Cardiac arrest >15 min without tissue perfusion
Frailty	Low	Moderate	High
Organ failure	Isolated respiratory failure	"Mild" additional organ failure	Severe acute multiorgan failure with anticipated death despite ECMO support
		Secondary infections with multidrug resistant organisms	
Mechanical ventilation	<7 days	>7 days	No agreed absolute contraindication
	High driving pressure > 15 cm H_2O	Unsuccessful trial of prone ventilation ≥6 h	
Scoring system		Indices of low potential to recover (e.g., a respiratory ECMO Survival Prediction [RESP] score of ≤ 3)	
Ethics	A declared or presumed patient's will in favour	Patient's will unclear, next of kin undecided	A declared or presumed patient's will against ECMO
System capacity	Normal/expanded capacity Normal/restricted criteria	Near saturation capacity Highly selective ECMO use only	Crisis capacity No further cannulations possible

Adapted from Badulak et al. [1], Dalia et al. [34], Camporota et al. [41], Karagiannidis et al. [40], and Herrmann et al. [44].

Table 2.
Selection criteria for VV ECMO in severe refractory COVID-19—A graduated approach.

ECMO support. Most participants stated that their criteria for starting ECMO had changed during the COVID-19 pandemic, with lower age limits, decreased ECMO machine availability, and stricter inclusion criteria. Interestingly, the majority of those surveyed agreed that it would be ethical to give extra priority to a healthcare worker who had contracted COVID-19 due to occupational exposure. Decision making pertaining to futility and cessation of therapy were predominantly guided by lack of benefit to the patient being supported, however, as the pandemic progressed, there was an increased move to a more utilitarian approach i.e., they would consider discontinuing ECMO in a patient with poor prognostic outcome, in order to provide ECMO to a patient more likely to survive [46]. The current ELSO guidance suggests that treatment may be regarded as futile and discontinued after 21 days. However, it is clear from the published data that COVID patients frequently require more prolonged ECMO support compared with other cohorts of up to 5 weeks duration [3, 47].

The process of patient selection is complex and multifactorial and for this reason optimal indications for ECMO support in patients with severe COVID-19 ARDS remain unknown. It is clear however that the indications for ECMO are moving away from rescue therapy and more into an extended form of standard conventional therapy.

Key points

- Patients with severe COVID-19 ARDS should be referred for ECMO early, preferably within the first week of mechanical ventilation.

- Age, ECMO centre experience, and concomitant disease are major risk factors for poor survival.

- Patient selection should be decided on a case-by-case basis guided by multiclinician shared decision making and careful assessment of several immunologic, biographic, medical, and prognostic parameters.

- ECMO in COVID-19 is time and resource-intensive, and not all patients will benefit from this invasive support. We have an ethical responsibility to select the right patient in order to avoid harm.

4. Outcomes in patients supported with VV ECMO during the COVID-19 pandemic

4.1 Predicting outcomes in ECMO and COVID ARDS

Prognostication in COVID ARDS patients being considered for ECMO is very challenging, particularly due to the inconsistent mortality data reported over the course of the pandemic. Various scoring systems have been suggested as an aid to improve risk stratification, prognostication, and allocation of resources, particularly when the healthcare system is constrained. These include the Respiratory ECMO Survival Prediction score (RESP) and the PRedicting dEath for SEvere ARDS on VV-ECMO (PRESERVE) score, both of which were developed exclusively for outcome prediction in patients requiring VV ECMO. Other scoring systems studied in ECMO patients include the Roch score, and general critical care scoring systems such as Sequential Organ Failure Assessment (SOFA) and SAPS II [48–50]. The RESP score was used by some centres during the pandemic to encourage shared decisions making amongst experts when faced with particularly high-risk challenging cases [41]. A prediction model development study by Moyon et al. demonstrated acceptable discrimination and a good calibration with the RESP score in comparison with both the PRESERVE score and more traditional critical care scores e.g., SOFA [51]. However, other studies have demonstrated poor predictive ability of all the above scoring systems, including the RESP score, with prognostic accuracy ranging between approximately 0.5 and 0.6 (based on the area under the receiver operating characteristic curve—AUROC) [52, 53]. The general consensus is that existing scoring tools appear to perform poorly in COVID-19 patients, both in terms of those being considered and those being supported with VV ECMO. They should not be used in isolation to guide patient selection or refusal, but should be applied judiciously, in conjunction with clinical judgement, expertise, and guideline recommendations.

4.2 Mortality

Initial case studies and case reports of VV ECMO in COVID-19 were discouraging. They suggested a high mortality and raised significant concerns regarding its potential use in this patient population [54–56]. However, as the pandemic evolved, subsequent ECMO COVID-19 outcome data published from the ELSO Registry reported an estimated cumulative incidence of 90-day in-hospital mortality of 37.4% (95% CI 34.4–40.4), comparable to outcomes after ECMO in non-COVID ARDS [30, 47]. This was supported by several other multicentre observational cohort studies [42, 57, 58]. One of these, a systematic review and meta-analysis by Ramanathan et al., examined the use of ECMO in adult patients with COVID-19 during the first year of the pandemic (Dec 2019 to Jan 2021). This included 22 observational studies, with 1896 patients included in the meta-analysis, and VV ECMO was used in 98.6% of cases. In-hospital mortality in patients receiving ECMO support for COVID-19 was 37.1% during the first year of the pandemic, similar to those with non-COVID-19-related ARDS [42].

As the pandemic progressed, mortality with VV ECMO utilisation in COVID-19 began to increase from the summer of 2020. Barbaro et al. demonstrated that prior to May 1st 2020, the COVID-19 ECMO mortality rate was 36.9% (95% CI 34.1–39.7) compared with 51.9% (50.0–53.8) for patients who started ECMO after this date. Mortality was even higher at 58.9% (55.4–62.3) for patients treated at centres that only offered ECMO after this date. This large multicentre retrospective study of 4812 patients broadly categorised patients as to whether they were managed at early adopting (groups A1 and A2) vs. late adopting centres (group B). Not only did they demonstrate a 15% increase in mortality over the course of the pandemic, but also an increase in the median duration of ECMO support by 6 days. Compared with to patients in group A2, group A1 patients had a lower adjusted relative risk of in-hospital mortality 90 days after ECMO (hazard ratio 0.82 [0.70–0.96]), whereas group B patients had a higher adjusted relative risk (1.42 [1.17–1.73]) [3]. The large multicentre French cohort study of the ECMOSARS registry data has one of the highest in-hospital mortality rates to date of 51%, although this may be due to several factors including an older population compared with the ELSO registry and STOP-COVID studies, a more severe COVID-ARDS phenotype (99% of patients met the Berlin definition criteria compared with 79% in the ELSO study, and a longer duration of mechanical ventilation before ECMO cannulation (median 6 days vs. 4 days in the ELSO study population) [47, 57, 59]. A meta-analysis of 6 studies by Bertini et al. found that the COVID-19 ECMO cohort had a 1.34 increased relative risk of mortality when compared to patients with influenza (44% vs. 38%; RR 1.34; 95% CI 1.05–1.71; $p = 0.03$) [60]. A robust systematic review and meta-analysis by Ling et al., which included a cohort of >18,000 COVID-19 patients receiving ECMO between Dec 2019 and Jan 2022, found a pooled mortality rate of 48.8%, higher than that reported in the review by Bertini et al. [27, 60].

However, other studies have shown more promising results. Shaefi and colleagues conducted an emulated target trial using observational data to assess the efficacy of ECMO compared with conventional mechanical ventilation in COVID-19. They included patients with severe hypoxemia and observed a reduction in mortality with ECMO (hazard ratio, 0.55; 95% confidence interval, 0.41–0.74) [57]. Urner et al. also performed an emulated target trial similar to Shaefi et al. They conducted a multicentre retrospective observational study of 7345 patients with severe COVID-ARDS admitted between January 2020 and August 2021, 844 of whom received VV ECMO support. They demonstrated a significant reduction in hospital mortality by 7.1% compared with conventional mechanical ventilation without ECMO. Secondary analyses revealed several factors that were significantly associated with reduced ECMO efficacy which are discussed below [61]. Most recently, Hajage et al. have added to the above emulated trial data with their multicentre observational cohort study of 2858 patients, 269 of whom were supported with ECMO. Overall survival at day 7 of ECMO support was high, and comparable between ECMO and non-ECMO survivors (87% vs. 83% respectively). Mortality increased as time progressed, with a reported survival rate of 63% at 90-days which was not significantly different to that of the conventional management group. However, they did demonstrate a significantly improved 90-day survival rate in high volume centres where ECMO was initiated early (within the first 4 days of intubation) in severe COVID ARDS; survival was 78% on ECMO vs. 64% in the conventional arm [4]. Finally, Whebell and colleagues also provided a more optimistic outlook in their multi-centre matched retrospective study of COVID-19 patients from 111 hospitals, referred to two specialist ECMO centres in the United Kingdom between March 2020 and February 2021 [62]. Of 1363 patients referred, 243 were retrieved on mobile ECMO to the quaternary centre. They demonstrated a marginal odds ratio (OR) for mortality of 0.44 (95% CI 0.29–0.68, $p < 0.001$) and absolute mortality reduction of 18.2% (44% vs. 25.8%, $p < 0.001$) for treatment with ECMO in a specialist centre, compared with patients managed conventionally in the referring hospital. The findings from Whebell et al. differ compared with other similar cohort studies. In their study, mortality did not increase significantly in the ECMO group during the second wave (22.9% vs. 26.1%, $p = 0.672$), however it increased significantly in those managed with conventional support (51.9% vs. 62.4%, $p = 0.001$). This is likely a factor of increased early adjunctive therapy e.g., immunomodulatory agents, and a greater implementation of more discerning ECMO selection criteria. Selected patients were also younger, with lower SOFA and higher RESP scores, and had less duration of organ support prior to ECMO. Notably, a higher proportion of patients with documented 'perceived futility' and a lower proportion of ECMO treated patients were seen in the second wave [62].

The variability in mortality seen in studies of ECMO support in COVID-19 patients to date is likely multifactorial (**Table 3**). Early studies were limited by the inclusion of unselected populations and the lack of adequate controls. In addition, there were substantial changes in the management of COVID-19 as the pandemic evolved, in line with rapidly emerging evidence from large multicentre platform studies, which may have affected the category of patient progressing to ECMO support [63–66]. Patients were frequently supported with high-flow oxygen, non-invasive ventilation, awake prone positioning, and immunomodulatory therapy as part of standard care which may have mitigated the need to advance to more invasive support therapy [67–73]. These developments occurred in parallel with a significant increase

Patient factors	Treatment factors	Organisational factors
Age ≥ 65	Pre-ECMO ventilatory therapy *duration, intensity *PaO2/ FiO2 ratio < 80 mmHg * DP >15cmH20	High volume centre experience
ARDS Phenotype		Time interval to ECMO i.e. symptoms to cannulation
		Cannula Fr size
≥ 2 Comorbidities * Hypertension * Obesity * Ischaemic heart disease * Diabetes	Refractory to ventilatory adjuncts *Proning *High PEEP *NMB * Inhaled pulmonary vasodilators	Duration of ECMO support Number of ECMO runs
Pulmonary hypertension +/− right ventricular dysfunction	Novel COVID-19 therapies *steroids *IL-6 inhibitors	
Male		

Table 3.
Summary of factors impacting mortality in COVID-19 patients supported with ECMO.

in the number of centres providing ECMO support to patients with COVID-19 [74]. In general, older age, increasing burden of comorbidity, increased vasopressor requirement and need for renal replacement therapy (RRT), and increased bleeding complications are more common in COVID-19 patients supported with ECMO who die compared with those who survive [75].

It is still unclear whether the use of VV ECMO definitively confers improved survival in patients with COVID-19 ARDS. Mortality rates and the duration of support required have so far been inconsistent. Different studies have shown variable outcomes for COVID-19 patients supported with VV ECMO depending on the phase of the pandemic [3]. Although Barbaro et al. reported a 90-day in-hospital mortality of 37% for COVID-19 patients supported with ECMO, we still do not know the long-term outcomes of COVID-19 ECMO patients who have survived [3, 47]. The most recent 60-day and 90-day ECMO survival data from the more recent emulated target trials is however very reassuring [4, 57, 61]. However, the findings from these studies must be taken in the context of certain limitations such as lack of random treatment allocation and unmeasured confounders which may have biased the study results in either direction [76].

4.3 Morbidity

Complications in critically ill patients receiving ECMO are well described, with higher incidence associated with longer duration of ECMO support, increased duration of mechanical ventilation, and coagulopathy associated with both pharmacotherapy and the prothrombotic environment within the ECMO circuit [47, 77–79]. The overall incidence of complications, in COVID-19 patients supported with ECMO (when defined as complication rates per 1000 hours of ECMO support), excluding renal replacement therapy, is 50–60%. Renal complications in general account for 10–30% overall, depending on the pandemic phase, definition/ parameters used, and other patient and treatment factors [3, 42].

Bleeding and thrombosis are common and are associated with increased mortality in patients supported with ECMO [80]. A retrospective ELSO registry study analysing bleeding and thrombotic events (BTEs) in 7579 VV-ECMO patients between 2010 and 2017, the largest multicentre study of its kind to date, reported a 40.2% incidence of ≥1 BTEs in patients supported with VV-ECMO. The in-hospital mortality rate associated with bleeding and/ or thrombosis was 34.9% in this cohort overall. Thrombotic events were more common than bleeding and comprised 54.9% of all BTEs. This contrasts with VA-ECMO where bleeding events tend to predominate [81]. The most common thrombotic events were circuit clotting (31.8%) and oxygenator/ pump failure (12.7%). Bleeding is common and complicates the course of approximately 16–60% of patients managed with ECMO [82, 83]. In the aforementioned ELSO registry study, cannulation sites (15.5%) and surgical bleeding (9.6%) were the most common sources, with medical bleeding accounting for 18.7% of events [80]. Intracranial haemorrhage was more common than ischemic stroke (4.5% vs. 1.9%, respectively). This is consistent with the findings from previous studies in this area, which have also reported incidences of other significant bleeding events such as gastrointestinal (5.5%) and pulmonary (6.1%) haemorrhage [82, 84]. Major bleeding requiring transfusion occurs in 39%, and the mortality associated with bleeding may be as high as 48.5% [85, 86]. The overall incidence of neurological complications in ECMO is approximately 7–9%, with intracranial haemorrhage accounting for 38% of these cases [87]. Of note, during the H1N1 influenza pandemic, intracerebral haemorrhage was reported as the commonest cause of death in patients supported with VV ECMO [88, 89].

Immune-mediated thrombosis has been postulated as a key mechanism in the pathophysiology of COVID-19, and its associated increased thrombotic risk profile. Much research has been dedicated to this area, and in finding the optimal anticoagulation strategy for these patients. However, there is little hard evidence to inform us of the specific bleeding and thrombosis risk in COVID-19 patients supported with ECMO. To date most of the evidence has come from case series reports. In the multicentre ECMOSARS cohort study of approximately 500 COVID-19 patients, haemorrhagic complications occurred in 40% patients, thrombosis occurred in 37%, and neurological complications in 11%. 80% of neurological complications were due to haemorrhagic stroke [59]. Interestingly, the incidence of haemorrhagic complications was higher compared with the Study of the Treatment and Outcomes in Critically Ill Patients with COVID-19 (STOP-COVID), 28% vs. 40%, and also that of the ELSO registry study [47, 57]. A follow-on ECMOSARS registry study by Mansour et al. analysed all patients in this registry over the course of the first and second pandemic waves from February 2020 to the end of March 2022 [90]. In this review, 65.5% of patients experienced either bleeding or thrombosis. Interestingly, thrombosis rates remained stable over the course of the pandemic (approximately 35%), while bleeding increased. Bleeding events (49% of patients) were associated with a significantly higher in-hospital 90-day mortality of 71.8%, unlike thrombosis which was not associated with a significantly increased mortality (adjOR = 1.02 [0.68–1.53]. The commonest bleeding and thrombosis sites were similiar to previous reported studies. Intracranial haemorrhage was independently associated with an increased mortality risk (adjOR = 13.5 [4.4–41.5]. Massive transfusion was required in 10% of bleeding events, and successive bleeding events increased mortality fourfold. Independent risk factors for bleeding included the duration of ECMO support and ventilation duration ≥7 days prior to ECMO cannulation, whilst a fibrinogen >6 g/ L at cannulation was predictive of thrombosis. Barbaro et al. reported similar rates of intracranial, pulmonary and gastrointestinal bleeding in their retrospective multicentre ELSO registry study, however the prevalence of cannula site bleeding events was lower (approximately 6% across the study subgroups) compared with the aforementioned ECMOSARS studies. In addition, they found that haemolytic, haemorrhagic, ischaemic, neurological, and mechanical complications were broadly similar in both early-adopting vs. late-adopting centres over the course of the pandemic [3]. The increased bleeding and lower thrombosis incidence reported by Mansour et al. compared with the ECMOSARS and Nunez et al. ELSO studies, particularly in relation to device thrombosis and membrane failure, is possibly related to the generalised augmentation of anticoagulation therapy over the course of the pandemic.

Notably, randomised controlled trials have not demonstrated a clear benefit for therapeutic heparin in critically ill patients with COVID-19. However, observational study data does suggest evidence of benefit for prophylactic dose low molecular weight heparin (LMWH) in non-critically ill COVID-19 patients in terms of organ support free days, even in those without a documented thrombotic event, albeit with an increased risk of bleeding, and this has formed the basis for widespread prophylactic anticoagulation in these patients [91, 92]. Despite increased knowledge of the risks of thrombosis and bleeding in immobilised COVID-19 patients supported with ECMO, the optimal anticoagulation regimen remains to be fully elucidated. There is no consensus on the optimal choice of anticoagulant, dosing, and duration of treatment; and there is significant regional and institutional variability in clinical practice. It becomes an even more complex scenario with the addition of ECMO, where a minimum threshold of systemic heparinisation and possibly antiplatelet cover are required to prevent circuit thrombosis. However, it is a double-edged sword, as ECMO also depletes host antithrombin (AT) levels through haemodilution, coagulation factor activation, and consumption by unfractionated heparin, thereby reducing heparin efficacy and potentially increasing the risk of thrombosis. Bleeding risk is also increased in AT depletion due to clotting factor consumption by the circuit, and also a relative increased inflammatory coagulopathic response due to a lack of AT anti-inflammatory activity [93]. To date, ELSO have not made any specific recommendations in this arena beyond usual recommended anticoagulation practice for patients receiving ECMO support [1].

Rates of infectious complications in COVID-19 patients on ECMO have been variable. The ECMOSARS Investigators demonstrated a much higher incidence of ventilator associated pneumonia (VAP) and bacteraemia of 51% and 41% respectively, compared with STOP-COVID (Study of the Treatment and Outcomes in Critically Ill Patients with COVID-19) which reported a 35% incidence of VAP and 18% incidence of other infections [57, 59]. This vulnerability to increased infection is likely multifactorial, related to the increased duration of mechanical ventilation, increased used of immunomodulatory agents e.g. steroids, IL-6 inhibitors etc., increased multidrug resistant organisms, and difficulties around maintaining sterility in a high stress and resource constrained environment. In the ECMOVIBER (The use of ECMO during the coVid-19 pandemic in the IBERian peninsula) study, co-infection at ECMO initiation was recorded in 29.8% of cases, although this was not significantly associated with increased mortality [43]. Unsurprisingly, the incidence of complications overall is significantly higher in non-survivors compared with survivors [59, 75].

4.4 Risk factors associated with morbidity and mortality

Age is the major factor predictive of increased mortality in COVID-ARDS patients supported with extracorporeal therapy, with age over 65 increasing mortality four-fold. The relationship between older age, defined in the ELSO guidelines as ≥65 years, and poorer survival is a constant finding in the COVID-19 literature, with OR doubling to 2.7 at 60–70 years and doubling again between 70 and 80 years [35, 94]. However, increasing age alone should not automatically exclude suitability for ECMO but should be reviewed in combination with pre-existing comorbidity and concomitant disease, including organ failure. A male preponderance, ≥2 comorbidities (particularly hypertension, diabetes, ischaemic heart disease, obesity, immunosuppression), the variant subtype, and a more severe ARDS phenotype with lack of reversibility are also associated with worse outcomes [3, 27, 58 , 59, 61, 75, 90]. Of note, there is some conflicting evidence to suggest that obesity is not associated with poorer outcomes in COVID ECMO patients, including increased 90-day mortality [95, 96].

As the pandemic evolved, the nature of pre-ECMO therapies also changed. The intensity and duration of these treatments may have impacted on morbidity and mortality in patients who went on to be supported with ECMO. For example, in the second wave compared with the first, there was a significant difference in the uptake of adjunctive therapies i.e., steroids 99.3% vs. 12%; IL-6 inhibitor 13.1% vs. 1%; NIV 78.2% vs. 49.6%; prone positioning 82.5% vs. 68.7%; and nitric oxide 16% vs. 6.1% [62]. In a recent systematic review and meta-analysis, most patients received neuromuscular blockade (96.2%) and were positioned prone (84.5%) prior to initiation of ECMO [42]. Many of these therapies have an established mortality benefit in COVID-19, steroids being the main example, and some patients may have a more responsive phenotype [97]. Therefore it is possible that the high mortality of approximately 40% in COVID ARDS patients supported with ECMO may stem from a selection bias for a more treatment resistant phenotype, given that patients who responded well to protective lung ventilation and adjunctive therapies may not have progressed to require ECMO. Immunomodulatory therapy may be associated with increased secondary infection, which may also have contributed to a worse ECMO survival rate [98].

The duration of mechanical ventilation pre cannulation has also been a topic of debate. Mechanical ventilation for longer than 7–10 days prior has traditionally been considered a contraindication to initiation of ECMO support as recommended in the 2017 and 2020 ELSO guidelines [35]. However, emerging evidence suggests that the duration of mechanical ventilation pre ECMO has no significant impact on mortality. It is actually the time interval from symptom onset to ECMO cannulation, and the driving pressure that are associated with a higher in-hospital mortality in this group [42, 43]. The comparative effectiveness of a PaO2/FiO2 ratio-guided vs. driving pressure guided ECMO initiation trigger has also been studied, with higher driving pressures at cannulation associated with poorer survival [43, 61]. The findings from a large registry study of approximately 7000 patients suggest that ECMO is possibly most effective if consistently provided to patients with more severe hypoxaemia i.e. PaO2/FiO2 < 80 mmHg, or driving pressure > 15 cm H_2O [61]. The relationship of mechanical ventilation therapy to ECMO survival may be influenced by the timing of intubation and IPPV (which tended to be early during the first wave compared with subsequent waves), and also as various non-invasive ventilation modalities e.g. high flow nasal cannula oxygen, CPAP, NIV etc., began to dominate the initial management phase of COVID ARDS.

COVID-19 patients require a prolonged duration of ECMO support compared with non-COVID ARDS to achieve successful weaning and ICU survival [30]. Approximately 25% of patients required at least 5 weeks or more of ECMO support [3, 47]. Interestingly, a longer duration of ECMO is not associated with increased mortality [27, 42]. This may be partly due to survival bias i.e., patients must survive a certain duration of time while supported with ECMO to fulfil the criteria for weaning, compared with other patients who may have had ECMO stopped earlier for futility or died [27, 42, 99]. Bridging to lung transplantation may also have skewed this data, as this would have removed some of the more critically unwell cohort who would probably not have survived without transplantation. However, studies reporting the use of lung transplantation in COVID-19 have so far been limited primarily to case reports and case series [100–102].

Organisational factors are also important to consider when examining mortality in COVID-19 patients supported with ECMO, especially given the heterogeneity across the major studies in relation to geographical, resource allocation, and temporal differences therein. A massive surge in capacity combined with a rapid upskilling of non-intensive care staff was required to deliver prompt and effective care to COVID-19 patients both in the main critical care ward and in non-critical care environments. Critical care surge capacity increased up to 155% in total, and 40% of COVID patients overall were managed in surge capacity beds. The patient to nurse ratio increased by about 25%, with most units requiring non-ICU clinicians and non-ICU nurses to aid with the increased workload (58% and 85% respectively). However, ECMO was generally employed only in the standard critical care bed setting [94]. Criteria for patient selection also varied over the course of the pandemic as knowledge of the disease evolved and as availability of resources changed [35]. Even now, ethical patient selection and timing of optimal ECMO initiation remains challenging.

High-volume ECMO centre experience, as measured by the number of ECMO runs greater than 30 per year, has a significant benefit on ICU mortality in COVID-ARDS [3, 44]. This was clearly demonstrated in the emulated target trial study by Hajage and colleagues where in high-volume experience centres, survival was 78% on ECMO vs. 64% for conventional management [4]. In other studies, survival in low vs. higher volume centres has been reported as 20% vs. 38% respectively [44]. The volume-survival relationship extends not only to those patients that receive ECMO support, but also those who are retrieved or transferred to the specialist high volume ECMO centre and do not receive ECMO. This has been demonstrated in non-COVID ARDS also [29]. Paradoxically, some healthcare systems demonstrated a higher in-hospital mortality across all phases of the pandemic despite being well resourced e.g. in Germany, there was an in-hospital mortality of about 70% over the entire pandemic, however this may be due to differences in patient selection criteria. The clinical and organisational factors associated with mortality in COVID-ARDS patients supported with ECMO are summarised in **Table 3**.

5. Conclusion

The COVID-19 pandemic has presented the most unparalleled global healthcare challenge since the influenza pandemic of 1918. Our knowledge of the disease and potentially efficacious therapy is constantly evolving, and yet patients with COVID ARDS remain at significantly increased risk of poor outcomes, including mortality. Although ECMO is a possible lifesaving option in those who are refractory to optimal conventional therapy, it is still unclear whether the use of VV ECMO definitively confers improved survival in patients with COVID-19 ARDS based on the mortality data thus far, although the more recent data is encouraging. We do know however, that improved survival depends on numerous factors, including resource allocation, patient selection criteria, timing of ECMO initiation, and centre volume experience. Judicious and ethical patient selection is therefore paramount to ensure the greatest benefit and least harm in the face of a constrained healthcare environment with finite resources.

Conflict of interest

No conflicts of interest to declare.

Author details

Cathal MacDonncha[1], Rachel Jooste[1], John Laffey[1,2,3] and Ciara Hanley[1,2]*

1 Department of Anaesthesia and Intensive Care Medicine, Galway University Hospitals, Saolta University Hospital Group, Galway, Ireland

2 School of Medicine, National University of Ireland, Galway, Ireland

3 Regenerative Medicine Institute, National University of Ireland, Galway, Ireland

*Address all correspondence to: CiaraM.Hanley@hse.ie

References

[1] Badulak J, Antonini MV, Stead CM, Shekerdemian L, Raman L, Paden ML, et al. Extracorporeal membrane oxygenation for COVID-19: Updated 2021 guidelines from the extracorporeal life support organization. ASAIO Journal. 2021;**67**(5):485-495

[2] Extracorporeal Life Support Organization E. Registry Dashboard of ECMO-Supported COVID-19 Patient Data. Available from: https://www.elso.org/Registry/FullCOVID-19RegistryDashboard.aspx

[3] Barbaro RP, MacLaren G, Boonstra PS, Combes A, Agerstrand C, Annich G, et al. Extracorporeal membrane oxygenation for COVID-19: Evolving outcomes from the international extracorporeal life support organization registry. Lancet. 2021;**398**(10307):1230-1238

[4] Hajage D, Combes A, Guervilly C, Lebreton G, Mercat A, Pavot A, et al. Extracorporeal membrane oxygenation for severe acute respiratory distress syndrome associated with COVID-19: An emulated target trial analysis. American Journal of Respiratory and Critical Care Medicine. 2022;**206**(3):281-294

[5] World Health Organisation. 2022. Available from: https://covid19.who.int/

[6] Force ADT, Ranieri VM, Rubenfeld GD, Thompson BT, Ferguson ND, Caldwell E, et al. Acute respiratory distress syndrome: The Berlin definition. Journal of the American Medical Association. 2012;**307**(23):2526-2533

[7] Camporota L, Ranieri VM. What's new in the "Berlin" definition of acute respiratory distress syndrome? Minerva Anestesiologica. 2012;**78**(10):1162-1166

[8] Camporota L, Cronin JN, Busana M, Gattinoni L, Formenti F. Pathophysiology of coronavirus-19 disease acute lung injury. Current Opinion in Critical Care. 2022;**28**(1):9-16

[9] de Roquetaillade C, Bredin S, Lascarrou JB, Soumagne T, Cojocaru M, Chousterman BG, et al. Timing and causes of death in severe COVID-19 patients. Critical Care. 2021;**25**(1):224

[10] Zhou F, Yu T, Du R, Fan G, Liu Y, Liu Z, et al. Clinical course and risk factors for mortality of adult inpatients with COVID-19 in Wuhan, China: A retrospective cohort study. Lancet. 2020;**395**(10229):1054-1062

[11] Carsana L, Sonzogni A, Nasr A, Rossi RS, Pellegrinelli A, Zerbi P, et al. Pulmonary post-mortem findings in a series of COVID-19 cases from northern Italy: A two-Centre descriptive study. The Lancet Infectious Diseases. 2020;**20**(10):1135-1140

[12] Menter T, Haslbauer JD, Nienhold R, Savic S, Hopfer H, Deigendesch N, et al. Postmortem examination of COVID-19 patients reveals diffuse alveolar damage with severe capillary congestion and variegated findings in lungs and other organs suggesting vascular dysfunction. Histopathology. 2020;**77**(2):198-209

[13] Schaller T, Hirschbuhl K, Burkhardt K, Braun G, Trepel M, Markl B, et al. Postmortem examination of patients with COVID-19. Journal of the American Medical Association. 2020;**323**(24):2518-2520

[14] Grasselli G, Tonetti T, Protti A, Langer T, Girardis M, Bellani G, et al. Pathophysiology of COVID-19-associated acute respiratory distress syndrome: A

multicentre prospective observational study. The Lancet Respiratory Medicine. 2020;**8**(12):1201-1208

[15] Panwar R, Madotto F, Laffey JG, van Haren FMP. Compliance phenotypes in early acute respiratory distress syndrome before the COVID-19 pandemic. American Journal of Respiratory and Critical Care Medicine. 2020;**202**(9):1244-1252

[16] Gattinoni L, Camporota L, Marini JJ. COVID-19 phenotypes: Leading or misleading? The European Respiratory Journal. 2020;**56**:2002195. DOI: 10.1183/13993003.02195-2020

[17] Gattinoni L, Chiumello D, Caironi P, Busana M, Romitti F, Brazzi L, et al. COVID-19 pneumonia: Different respiratory treatments for different phenotypes? Intensive Care Medicine. 2020;**46**(6):1099-1102

[18] Gattinoni L, Chiumello D, Rossi S. COVID-19 pneumonia: ARDS or not? Critical Care. 2020;**24**(1):154

[19] Maiolo G, Collino F, Vasques F, Rapetti F, Tonetti T, Romitti F, et al. Reclassifying acute respiratory distress syndrome. American Journal of Respiratory and Critical Care Medicine. 2018;**197**(12):1586-1595

[20] Camporota L, Vasques F, Sanderson B, Barrett NA, Gattinoni L. Identification of pathophysiological patterns for triage and respiratory support in COVID-19. The Lancet Respiratory Medicine. 2020;**8**(8):752-754

[21] Vandenbunder B, Ehrmann S, Piagnerelli M, Sauneuf B, Serck N, Soumagne T, et al. Static compliance of the respiratory system in COVID-19 related ARDS: An international multicenter study. Critical Care. 2021;**25**(1):52

[22] Ferrando C, Suarez-Sipmann F, Mellado-Artigas R, Hernández M, Gea A, Arruti E, et al. Clinical features, ventilatory management, and outcome of ARDS caused by COVID-19 are similar to other causes of ARDS. Intensive Care Medicine. 2020;**46**(12):2200-2211

[23] Boscolo A, Sella N, Lorenzoni G, Pettenuzzo T, Pasin L, Pretto C, et al. Static compliance and driving pressure are associated with ICU mortality in intubated COVID-19 ARDS. Critical Care. 2021;**25**(1):263

[24] Paternoster G, Bertini P, Innelli P, Trambaiolo P, Landoni G, Franchi F, et al. Right ventricular dysfunction in patients with COVID-19: A systematic review and meta-analysis. Journal of Cardiothoracic and Vascular Anesthesia. 2021;**35**(11):3319-3324

[25] Reis Miranda D, van Thiel R, Brodie D, Bakker J. Right ventricular unloading after initiation of venovenous extracorporeal membrane oxygenation. American Journal of Respiratory and Critical Care Medicine. 2015;**191**(3):346-348

[26] Gattinoni L, Gattarello S, Steinberg I, Busana M, Palermo P, Lazzari S, et al. COVID-19 pneumonia: Pathophysiology and management. European Respiratory Review. 2021;**30**:210138. DOI: 10.1183/16000617.0138-2021

[27] Ling RR, Ramanathan K, Sim JJL, Wong SN, Chen Y, Amin F, et al. Evolving outcomes of extracorporeal membrane oxygenation during the first 2 years of the COVID-19 pandemic: A systematic review and meta-analysis. Critical Care. 2022;**26**(1):147

[28] Chow J, Alhussaini A, Calvillo-Arguelles O, Billia F, Luk A. Cardiovascular collapse in COVID-19 infection: The role of venoarterial extracorporeal membrane

oxygenation (VA-ECMO). CJC Open. 2020;**2**(4):273-277

[29] Peek GJ, Mugford M, Tiruvoipati R, Wilson A, Allen E, Thalanany MM, et al. Efficacy and economic assessment of conventional ventilatory support versus extracorporeal membrane oxygenation for severe adult respiratory failure (CESAR): A multicentre randomised controlled trial. Lancet. 2009;**374**(9698):1351-1363

[30] Combes A, Hajage D, Capellier G, Demoule A, Lavoue S, Guervilly C, et al. Extracorporeal membrane oxygenation for severe acute respiratory distress syndrome. The New England Journal of Medicine. 2018;**378**(21):1965-1975

[31] Zapol WM, Snider MT, Hill JD, Fallat RJ, Bartlett RH, Edmunds LH, et al. Extracorporeal membrane oxygenation in severe acute respiratory failure. A randomized prospective study. JAMA. 1979;**242**(20):2193-2196

[32] Morris AH, Wallace CJ, Menlove RL, Clemmer TP, Orme JF Jr, Weaver LK, et al. Randomized clinical trial of pressure-controlled inverse ratio ventilation and extracorporeal CO2 removal for adult respiratory distress syndrome. American Journal of Respiratory and Critical Care Medicine. 1994;**149**(2 Pt 1):295-305

[33] Combes A, Peek GJ, Hajage D, Hardy P, Abrams D, Schmidt M, et al. ECMO for severe ARDS: Systematic review and individual patient data meta-analysis. Intensive Care Medicine. 2020;**46**(11):2048-2057

[34] Dalia AA, Convissar D, Crowley J, Raz Y, Funamoto M, Wiener-Kronish J, et al. The role of extracorporeal membrane oxygenation in COVID-19. Journal of Cardiothoracic and Vascular Anesthesia. Sep 2022;**36**(9):3668-3675. DOI: 10.1053/j.jvca.2022.05.010

[35] Shekar K, Badulak J, Peek G, Boeken U, Dalton HJ, Arora L, et al. Extracorporeal life support organization coronavirus disease 2019 interim guidelines: A consensus document from an International Group of Interdisciplinary Extracorporeal Membrane Oxygenation Providers. ASAIO Journal. 2020;**66**(7):707-721

[36] Enforcement Policy for Extracorporeal Membrane Oxygenation and Cardiopulmonary Bypass Devices During the Coronavirus Disease 2019 (COVID-19) Public Health Emergency. In: U.S. Food and Drug Administration CfDaRH, Office of Product Evaluation and Quality, editor. 2020

[37] WHO WHO. Clinical Management of COVID-19: Living Guideline. 2022. Available from: https://files.magicapp.org/guideline/b487d134-4901-48a4-b145-d1a367ebbbdf/published_guideline_6470-4_1.pdf

[38] Alhazzani W, Moller MH, Arabi YM, Loeb M, Gong MN, Fan E, et al. Surviving sepsis campaign: Guidelines on the management of critically ill adults with coronavirus disease 2019 (COVID-19). Critical Care Medicine. 2020;**48**(6):e440-ee69

[39] Ramanathan K, Antognini D, Combes A, Paden M, Zakhary B, Ogino M, et al. Planning and provision of ECMO services for severe ARDS during the COVID-19 pandemic and other outbreaks of emerging infectious diseases. The Lancet Respiratory Medicine. 2020;**8**(5):518-526

[40] Karagiannidis C, Bein T, Welte T. ECMO during the COVID-19 pandemic: Moving from rescue therapy to more reasonable indications.

The European Respiratory Journal. 10 Feb 2022;**59**(2):2103262. DOI: 10.1183/13993003.03262-2021

[41] Camporota L, Meadows C, Ledot S, Scott I, Harvey C, Garcia M, et al. Consensus on the referral and admission of patients with severe respiratory failure to the NHS ECMO service. The Lancet Respiratory Medicine. 2021;**9**(2):e16-ee7

[42] Ramanathan K, Shekar K, Ling RR, Barbaro RP, Wong SN, Tan CS, et al. Extracorporeal membrane oxygenation for COVID-19: A systematic review and meta-analysis. Critical Care. 2021;**25**(1):211

[43] Riera J, Alcantara S, Bonilla C, Fortuna P, Blandino Ortiz A, Vaz A, et al. Risk factors for mortality in patients with COVID-19 needing extracorporeal respiratory support. The European Respiratory Journal. 10 Feb 2022;**59**(2):2102463. DOI: 10.1183/13993003.02463-2021

[44] Herrmann J, Lotz C, Karagiannidis C, Weber-Carstens S, Kluge S, Putensen C, et al. Key characteristics impacting survival of COVID-19 extracorporeal membrane oxygenation. Critical Care. 2022;**26**(1):190

[45] Bartlett RH, Ogino MT, Brodie D, McMullan DM, Lorusso R, MacLaren G, et al. Initial ELSO guidance document: ECMO for COVID-19 patients with severe cardiopulmonary failure. ASAIO Journal. 2020;**66**(5):472-474

[46] Dao B, Savulescu J, Suen JY, Fraser JF, Wilkinson DJC. Ethical factors determining ECMO allocation during the COVID-19 pandemic. BMC Medical Ethics. 2021;**22**(1):70

[47] Barbaro RP, MacLaren G, Boonstra PS, Iwashyna TJ, Slutsky AS, Fan E, et al. Extracorporeal membrane oxygenation support in COVID-19: An international cohort study of the extracorporeal life support organization registry. Lancet. 2020;**396**(10257):1071-1078

[48] Schmidt M, Zogheib E, Roze H, Repesse X, Lebreton G, Luyt CE, et al. The PRESERVE mortality risk score and analysis of long-term outcomes after extracorporeal membrane oxygenation for severe acute respiratory distress syndrome. Intensive Care Medicine. 2013;**39**(10):1704-1713

[49] Schmidt M, Bailey M, Sheldrake J, Hodgson C, Aubron C, Rycus PT, et al. Predicting survival after extracorporeal membrane oxygenation for severe acute respiratory failure. The respiratory extracorporeal membrane oxygenation survival prediction (RESP) score. American Journal of Respiratory and Critical Care Medicine. 2014;**189**(11):1374-1382

[50] Roch A, Hraiech S, Masson E, Grisoli D, Forel JM, Boucekine M, et al. Outcome of acute respiratory distress syndrome patients treated with extracorporeal membrane oxygenation and brought to a referral center. Intensive Care Medicine. 2014;**40**(1):74-83

[51] Moyon Q, Pineton de Chambrun M, Lebreton G, Chaieb H, Combes A, Schmidt M. Validation of survival prediction models for ECMO in Sars-CoV-2-related acute respiratory distress syndrome. Critical Care. 2022;**26**(1):187

[52] Supady A, DellaVolpe J, Taccone FS, Scharpf D, Ulmer M, Lepper PM, et al. Outcome prediction in patients with severe COVID-19 requiring extracorporeal membrane oxygenation—A retrospective international multicenter study.

Membranes (Basel). 2021;**11**(3):170. DOI: 10.3390/membranes11030170

[53] Gannon WD, Stokes JW, Gong W, Lindsell CJ, Tonna JE, Bacchetta M, et al. Predicting mortality for patients eligible for extracorporeal membrane oxygenation for COVID-19. American Journal of Respiratory and Critical Care Medicine. 1 Sep 2022;1;**206**(5):628-632. DOI: 10.1164/rccm.202202-0237LE

[54] Yang X, Cai S, Luo Y, Zhu F, Hu M, Zhao Y, et al. Extracorporeal membrane oxygenation for coronavirus disease 2019-induced acute respiratory distress syndrome: A multicenter descriptive study. Critical Care Medicine. 2020;**48**(9):1289-1295

[55] Zeng Y, Cai Z, Xianyu Y, Yang BX, Song T, Yan Q. Prognosis when using extracorporeal membrane oxygenation (ECMO) for critically ill COVID-19 patients in China: A retrospective case series. Critical Care. 2020;**24**(1):148

[56] Henry BM, Lippi G. Poor survival with extracorporeal membrane oxygenation in acute respiratory distress syndrome (ARDS) due to coronavirus disease 2019 (COVID-19): Pooled analysis of early reports. Journal of Critical Care. 2020;**58**:27-28

[57] Shaefi S, Brenner SK, Gupta S, O'Gara BP, Krajewski ML, Charytan DM, et al. Extracorporeal membrane oxygenation in patients with severe respiratory failure from COVID-19. Intensive Care Medicine. 2021;**47**(2): 208-221

[58] Schmidt M, Hajage D, Lebreton G, Monsel A, Voiriot G, Levy D, et al. Extracorporeal membrane oxygenation for severe acute respiratory distress syndrome associated with COVID-19: A retrospective cohort study. The Lancet Respiratory Medicine. 2020;**8**(11):1121-1131

[59] Nesseler N, Fadel G, Mansour A, Para M, Falcoz PE, Mongardon N, et al. Extracorporeal membrane oxygenation for respiratory failure related to COVID-19: A nationwide cohort study. Anesthesiology. 2022;**136**(5):732-748

[60] Bertini P, Guarracino F, Falcone M, Nardelli P, Landoni G, Nocci M, et al. ECMO in COVID-19 patients: A systematic review and meta-analysis. Journal of Cardiothoracic and Vascular Anesthesia. 2022;**36**(8 Pt A):2700-2706

[61] Urner M, Barnett AG, Bassi GL, Brodie D, Dalton HJ, Ferguson ND, et al. Venovenous extracorporeal membrane oxygenation in patients with acute covid-19 associated respiratory failure: Comparative effectiveness study. BMJ. 2022;**377**:e068723

[62] Whebell S, Zhang J, Lewis R, Berry M, Ledot S, Retter A, et al. Survival benefit of extracorporeal membrane oxygenation in severe COVID-19: A multi-centre-matched cohort study. Intensive Care Medicine. 2022;**48**(4):467-478

[63] Group RC, Horby P, Lim WS, Emberson JR, Mafham M, Bell JL, et al. Dexamethasone in hospitalized patients with Covid-19. The New England Journal of Medicine. 2021;**384**(8):693-704

[64] Beigel JH, Tomashek KM, Dodd LE, Mehta AK, Zingman BS, Kalil AC, et al. Remdesivir for the treatment of Covid-19—final report. The New England Journal of Medicine. 2020;**383**(19):1813-1826

[65] Hermine O, Mariette X, Tharaux PL, Resche-Rigon M, Porcher R, Ravaud P, et al. Effect of tocilizumab vs usual care in adults hospitalized with COVID-19

and moderate or severe pneumonia: A randomized clinical trial. JAMA Internal Medicine. 2021;**181**(1):32-40

[66] Angus DC, Derde L, Al-Beidh F, Annane D, Arabi Y, Beane A, et al. Effect of hydrocortisone on mortality and organ support in patients with severe COVID-19: The REMAP-CAP COVID-19 corticosteroid domain randomized clinical trial. Journal of the American Medical Association. 2020;**324**(13):1317-1329

[67] Beran A, Srour O, Malhas SE, Mhanna M, Ayesh H, Sajdeya O, et al. High-flow nasal cannula oxygen versus non-invasive ventilation in subjects with COVID-19: A systematic review and meta-analysis of comparative studies. Respiratory Care. Sep 2022;**67**(9):1177-1189. DOI: 10.4187/respcare.09987

[68] Bertaina M, Nunez-Gil IJ, Franchin L, Fernandez Rozas I, Arroyo-Espliguero R, Viana-Llamas MC, et al. Non-invasive ventilation for SARS-CoV-2 acute respiratory failure: A subanalysis from the HOPE COVID-19 registry. Emergency Medicine Journal. 2021;**38**(5):359-365

[69] Ospina-Tascon GA, Calderon-Tapia LE, Garcia AF, Zarama V, Gomez-Alvarez F, Alvarez-Saa T, et al. Effect of high-flow oxygen therapy vs conventional oxygen therapy on invasive mechanical ventilation and clinical recovery in patients with severe COVID-19: A randomized clinical trial. Journal of the American Medical Association. 2021;**326**(21):2161-2171

[70] Grieco DL, Menga LS, Cesarano M, Rosa T, Spadaro S, Bitondo MM, et al. Effect of helmet noninvasive ventilation vs high-flow nasal oxygen on days free of respiratory support in patients with COVID-19 and moderate to severe hypoxemic respiratory failure: The HENIVOT randomized clinical trial. Journal of the American Medical Association. 2021;**325**(17):1731-1743

[71] Li J, Luo J, Pavlov I, Perez Y, Tan W, Roca O, et al. Awake prone positioning for non-intubated patients with COVID-19-related acute hypoxaemic respiratory failure: A systematic review and meta-analysis. The Lancet Respiratory Medicine. 2022;**10**(6):573-583

[72] Pavlov I, He H, McNicholas B, Perez Y, Tavernier E, Trump MW, et al. Awake prone positioning in non-intubated patients with acute hypoxemic respiratory failure due to COVID-19. Respiratory Care. Jan 2022;**67**(1):102-114. DOI: 10.4187/respcare.09191

[73] Ehrmann S, Li J, Ibarra-Estrada M, Perez Y, Pavlov I, McNicholas B, et al. Awake prone positioning for COVID-19 acute hypoxaemic respiratory failure: A randomised, controlled, multinational, open-label meta-trial. The Lancet Respiratory Medicine. 2021;**9**(12):1387-1395

[74] Lorusso R, Combes A, Lo Coco V, De Piero ME, Belohlavek J, Euro EC-W, et al. ECMO for COVID-19 patients in Europe and Israel. Intensive Care Medicine. 2021;**47**(3):344-348

[75] Chong WH, Saha BK, Medarov BI. Clinical characteristics between survivors and nonsurvivors of COVID-19 patients requiring extracorporeal membrane oxygenation (ECMO) support: A systematic review and meta-analysis. Journal of Intensive Care Medicine. 2022;**37**(3):304-318

[76] Ferreyro BL, Fan E. Turning the page on extracorporeal membrane oxygenation for acute respiratory distress syndrome due to severe COVID-19. American Journal of

Respiratory and Critical Care Medicine. 2022;**206**(3):236-239

[77] Suh YJ, Hong H, Ohana M, Bompard F, Revel MP, Valle C, et al. Pulmonary embolism and deep vein thrombosis in COVID-19: A systematic review and meta-analysis. Radiology. 2021;**298**(2):E70-E80

[78] Luyt CE, Sahnoun T, Gautier M, Vidal P, Burrel S, Pineton de Chambrun M, et al. Ventilator-associated pneumonia in patients with SARS-CoV-2-associated acute respiratory distress syndrome requiring ECMO: A retrospective cohort study. Annals of Intensive Care. 2020;**10**(1):158

[79] Kannapadi NV, Jami M, Premraj L, Etchill EW, Giuliano K, Bush EL, et al. Neurological complications in COVID-19 patients with ECMO support: A systematic review and meta-analysis. Heart, Lung & Circulation. 2022;**31**(2):292-298

[80] Nunez JI, Gosling AF, O'Gara B, Kennedy KF, Rycus P, Abrams D, et al. Bleeding and thrombotic events in adults supported with venovenous extracorporeal membrane oxygenation: An ELSO registry analysis. Intensive Care Medicine. 2022;**48**(2):213-224

[81] Chung M, Cabezas FR, Nunez JI, Kennedy KF, Rick K, Rycus P, et al. Hemocompatibility-related adverse events and survival on venoarterial extracorporeal life support: An ELSO registry analysis. JACC: Heart Failure. 2020;**8**(11):892-902

[82] Mazzeffi M, Greenwood J, Tanaka K, Menaker J, Rector R, Herr D, et al. Bleeding, transfusion, and mortality on extracorporeal life support: ECLS working group on thrombosis and hemostasis. The Annals of Thoracic Surgery. 2016;**101**(2):682-689

[83] Vaquer S, de Haro C, Peruga P, Oliva JC, Artigas A. Systematic review and meta-analysis of complications and mortality of veno-venous extracorporeal membrane oxygenation for refractory acute respiratory distress syndrome. Annals of Intensive Care. 2017;**7**(1):51

[84] Thiagarajan RR, Barbaro RP, Rycus PT, McMullan DM, Conrad SA, Fortenberry JD, et al. Extracorporeal life support organization registry international report 2016. ASAIO Journal. 2017;**63**(1):60-67

[85] Lebreton G, Schmidt M, Ponnaiah M, Folliguet T, Para M, Guihaire J, et al. Extracorporeal membrane oxygenation network organisation and clinical outcomes during the COVID-19 pandemic in greater Paris, France: A multicentre cohort study. The Lancet Respiratory Medicine. 2021;**9**(8):851-862

[86] Ried M, Sommerauer L, Lubnow M, Muller T, Philipp A, Lunz D, et al. Thoracic bleeding complications in patients with Venovenous extracorporeal membrane oxygenation. The Annals of Thoracic Surgery. 2018;**106**(6):1668-1674

[87] Akoumianaki E, Jonkman A, Sklar MC, Georgopoulos D, Brochard L. A rational approach on the use of extracorporeal membrane oxygenation in severe hypoxemia: Advanced technology is not a panacea. Annals of Intensive Care. 2021;**11**(1):107

[88] Australia, New Zealand Extracorporeal Membrane Oxygenation Influenza I, Davies A, Jones D, Bailey M, Beca J, et al. Extracorporeal membrane oxygenation for 2009 influenza A(H1N1) acute respiratory distress syndrome. Journal of the American Medical Association. 2009;**302**(17):1888-1895

[89] Luyt CE, Brechot N, Demondion P, Jovanovic T, Hekimian G, Lebreton G,

et al. Brain injury during venovenous extracorporeal membrane oxygenation. Intensive Care Medicine. 2016;**42**(5):897-907

[90] Mansour A, Flecher E, Schmidt M, Rozec B, Gouin-Thibault I, Esvan M, et al. Bleeding and thrombotic events in patients with severe COVID-19 supported with extracorporeal membrane oxygenation: A nationwide cohort study. Intensive Care Medicine. Aug 2022;**48**(8):1039-1052. DOI: 10.1007/s00134-022-06794-y

[91] Cuker A, Tseng EK, Nieuwlaat R, Angchaisuksiri P, Blair C, Dane K, et al. American Society of Hematology 2021 guidelines on the use of anticoagulation for thromboprophylaxis in patients with COVID-19. Blood Advances. 2021;**5**(3):872-888

[92] Cuker A, Tseng EK, Schunemann HJ, Angchaisuksiri P, Blair C, Dane K, et al. American Society of Hematology living guidelines on the use of anticoagulation for thromboprophylaxis in patients with COVID-19: March 2022 update on the use of anticoagulation in critically ill patients. Blood Advances. 13 Sep 2022;**6**(17):4975-4982. DOI: 10.1182/bloodadvances.2022007940

[93] Kowalewski M, Fina D, Slomka A, Raffa GM, Martucci G, Lo Coco V, et al. COVID-19 and ECMO: The interplay between coagulation and inflammation-a narrative review. Critical Care. 2020;**24**(1):205

[94] Greco M, De Corte T, Ercole A, Antonelli M, Azoulay E, Citerio G, et al. Clinical and organizational factors associated with mortality during the peak of first COVID-19 wave: The global UNITE-COVID study. Intensive Care Medicine. 2022;**48**(6):690-705

[95] Daviet F, Guilloux P, Hraiech S, Tonon D, Velly L, Bourenne J, et al. Impact of obesity on survival in COVID-19 ARDS patients receiving ECMO: Results from an ambispective observational cohort. Annals of Intensive Care. 2021;**11**(1):157

[96] Galvagno SM Jr, Pelekhaty S, Cornachione CR, Deatrick KB, Mazzeffi MA, Scalea TM, et al. Does weight matter? Outcomes in adult patients on venovenous extracorporeal membrane oxygenation when stratified by obesity class. Anesthesia and Analgesia. 2020;**131**(3):754-761

[97] Chaudhuri D, Sasaki K, Karkar A, Sharif S, Lewis K, Mammen MJ, et al. Corticosteroids in COVID-19 and non-COVID-19 ARDS: A systematic review and meta-analysis. Intensive Care Medicine. 2021;**47**(5):521-537

[98] Gangneux JP, Dannaoui E, Fekkar A, Luyt CE, Botterel F, De Prost N, et al. Fungal infections in mechanically ventilated patients with COVID-19 during the first wave: The French multicentre MYCOVID study. The Lancet Respiratory Medicine. 2022;**10**(2):180-190

[99] Poon WH, Ramanathan K, Ling RR, Yang IX, Tan CS, Schmidt M, et al. Prone positioning during venovenous extracorporeal membrane oxygenation for acute respiratory distress syndrome: A systematic review and meta-analysis. Critical Care. 2021;**25**(1):292

[100] Bharat A, Querrey M, Markov NS, Kim S, Kurihara C, Garza-Castillon R, et al. Lung transplantation for patients with severe COVID-19. Science Translational Medicine. 16 Dec 2020;**12**(574)

[101] Lang C, Jaksch P, Hoda MA, Lang G, Staudinger T, Tschernko E,

et al. Lung transplantation for COVID-19-associated acute respiratory distress syndrome in a PCR-positive patient. The Lancet Respiratory Medicine. 2020;**8**(10):1057-1060

[102] Urlik M, Szuldrzynski K, Stacel T, Necki M, Bielanski P, Jankowski M, et al. First lung transplantation as a treatment of a patient supported with extracorporeal membrane oxygenation (ECMO) after COVID-19 in Poland. Advances in Respiratory Medicine. 2021;**89**(3):328-333

Chapter 11

ECMO Predictive Scores, Past, Present, and Future

Neel Shah and Ahmed Said

Abstract

Over the five decades since the first successful reports of extracorporeal membrane oxygenation (ECMO) use, ideal patient selection has been an ongoing question. This has led to the development of several prognostication tools aimed at identifying risk factors associated with poor outcomes. These have spanned neonatal, pediatric and adult patients supported on ECMO for cardiac or respiratory failure. The majority of these scores have focused on mortality as an objective poor outcome with only 2 adult scores looking at long-term neuropsychological outcomes in ECMO survivors. In the development of these scores the authors have mainly relied on registry style data with limited granularity and focused on immediate pre-ECMO data points without incorporation of the evolving patient trajectories leading up to ECMO cannulation. While such scores can be useful in both prognostication and as risk stratification and quality assessment tools, they all lack practicality on an individual patient level with regards to decision making, as these scores have all been developed on data from patients already supported on ECMO without a comparable control cohort, to truly mimic decision making at the bedside. In this chapter we review the currently available ECMO prognostication scores, their limitations and potential future directions.

Keywords: ECMO, predictive scores, mortality, predictive analytics, machine learning

1. Introduction

Throughout the history of extracorporeal membrane oxygenation (ECMO) from the first reported successful use in an adult patient in 1972 [1] and subsequently in neonates with respiratory failure [2], and then followed by the exponential increased use in adults following the CESAR trial [3], there has been interest in identifying patients who would benefit most from this high-risk resource-intensive therapy. Early efforts focused on using predictive scores of severe neonatal respiratory failure [4]; Newborn Pulmonary Insufficiency Index (a score developed by plotting serial inspired oxygen values with serial pH measurements in the first 24 hours of life) [5] and serial alveolar-arterial oxygen gradients (A-a DO2) [6], were deployed with mixed results. Since then, there have been extensive efforts at developing tools to aid in early identification of patients who would benefit most from timely institution of ECMO support and those with a high risk of mortality while being supported by ECMO. In this chapter, we provide a review of the currently available ECMO prediction tools, their development, validation and limitations and an outline of potential future directions of ECMO decision support tools.

2. ECMO outcomes prediction scores to date

The need for predictive scoring algorithms is particularly vital with deployment of a high resource therapy like extracorporeal life support. Over the last several decades various groups have published predictive scores typically focusing on mortality, with the hope to help guide clinical decision making for optimal patient selection prior to cannulation, and often to help stratify patient risk. The overall goal being to help identify patients most likely to benefit, and these scores have ranged in accuracy (measured by the Area Under the Receiver Operative Curve) from 0.65 to 0.89 [7].

To date, these scores have been focused on the broad pathophysiology of the disease necessitating ECMO support; respiratory failure requiring veno-venous (VV) ECMO and cardiac failure necessitating support by veno-arterial (VA) ECMO.

2.1 Respiratory failure

2.1.1 Neonatal - congenital diaphragmatic hernia

Congenital diaphragmatic hernia (CDH) continues to be one of the most common reasons for ECMO use in the neonatal age group [8]. This unique pathology is characterized by a failure of diaphragmatic development, associated lung hypoplasia and subsequent persistent pulmonary hypertension of the newborn (PPHN) and as such typically presents with isolated refractory respiratory or combined respiratory and cardiac failure shortly after birth [9].

As worsening hypoxia and hypercapnia after birth often exacerbate pulmonary hypertension in turn leading to worsening gas exchange and hemodynamics, the potential need exists for ECMO as a rescue therapy for those with severe CDH [9]. Prediction of CDH severity is often identified prenatally and is based off genetic testing, the sidedness of the CDH, liver position (proportion in the thorax), and observed to expected fetal lung volume by magnetic resonance imaging (MRI) [10]. Despite decades-long use of ECMO for CDH, there continue to ongoing controversies surrounding ECMO use in this unique population. Outcomes remain variable, controversy exists regarding if the optimal support modality is VV or VA ECMO and the timing of ECMO initiation, as well as if surgical repair is best performed early or late and finally if surgical repair should be performed while on ECMO support due to the increased possibility of associated bleeding complications [11–14]. The CDH working groups for both the Extracorporeal Life Support Organization (ELSO) and its European chapter (EuroELSO) have published entry criteria for utilizing severity of hypoxemia, impaired ventilation and impaired tissue perfusion prior to ECMO as indications and prematurity, weight, comorbidities and duration of mechanical ventilation as relative contraindications [15–17].

Currently two CDH ECMO specific mortality risk prediction models exist utilizing data from the ELSO registry data from 2000 to 2015, including over 4000 ECMO supported neonates [18]. Using multivariable logistic regression analyses using both complete data sets and 10 imputed data sets, the authors developed two predictive models, a pre-ECMO mortality risk score and another on-ECMO mortality risk score.

By dividing the studied cohort into a two thirds development cohort and a one third validation cohort, the authors included pre-ECMO ventilatory settings and adequacy of gas exchange as measured by blood pH in addition to CDH specific risk factors including CDH sidedness and repair on ECMO. The developed pre-ECMO model performed modestly with C statistics of 0.65. With the addition of on-ECMO complications; neurologic, renal and infectious, the on-ECMO Prediction model performance improved to C = 0.73 (**Table 1**). The authors recognized the value of these models specifically in research and quality improvement projects with cautious application in patient management.

2.1.2 Neonatal

Two commonly utilized scores exist to predict ECMO mortality risk in the general neonatal population beyond CDH.

The Pittsburgh Index for Pre-ECMO Risk (PIPER) was developed utilizing 5455 neonatal respiratory VA-ECMO patients from the ELSO registry from 2000 to 2010 to predict survival to hospital discharge [19]. PIPER was developed on seven pre-ECMO variables including patient characteristics; age, weight and the diagnosis of CDH in addition to markers of hemodynamic compromise and severity of respiratory failure prior to ECMO initiation; mean arterial blood pressure (MAP), pH, partial pressure of oxygen (pO_2) and use of inhaled nitric oxide (iNO). The authors found that each increasing quartile had a 15% increased risk of mortality. Despite the focus on pre-ECMO risk, the authors also conducted further modeling to include on-ECMO variables such as ECMO duration and complications (hemorrhagic, mechanical, neurologic, pulmonary and renal), which increased the predictive power of the PIPER model from an area under the receiver operator curve (AUROC) of 0.74 to 0.79. While not developed to focus only on CDH patients, CDH was much more common in the highest PIPER quartiles. Older age at ECMO initiation was also found to be associated with decreased survival [19].

The Neonatal Risk Estimate Score for Children Using Extracorporeal Respiratory Support (Neo-RESCUERs) was similarly designed to predict mortality for neonates receiving ECMO respiratory support [20]. It was developed and validated on 4592 neonates in the ELSO registry between 2008 and 2013, with January 1st 2012 as the cutoff date between the initial derivation cohort and the subsequent internal validation dataset. Validation was performed on patients with complete data in addition to those with imputed data. The investigators included patient demographics (age, gestational age, birth weight, sex, diagnosis), markers of respiratory and cardiac failure (pH, partial pressure of carbon dioxide ($PaCO_2$), ratio of arterial partial pressure of oxygen to fraction of inspired oxygen (PF ratio), oxygenation index (OI), and history of cardiac arrest) in addition to renal failure and comorbid conditions prior to ECMO cannulation (**Table 1**). They demonstrated their lowest decile having a predicted mortality of 4.4% compared to an observed mortality of 7%, and their highest decile having a predicted mortality of 67.5% and observed mortality of 65.6%. CDH in this group had 11-fold higher adjusted odds for mortality compared to meconium aspiration, pre-ECMO renal failure also had a much higher odds of mortality. As is the case with similar registry-based scores, the authors acknowledge the significant limitations with reliance on only the available variables in addition to the retrospective nature of the study and the inclusion of only ECMO supported patients. As such, they recommend the use of Neo-RESCUERS as a benchmarking and risk stratification tool rather than an ECMO decision support tool.

Score	Year	Variables	Patient cohort
CDH Pre-ECMO	2018	Prior CDH repair Critical congenital heart disease Perinatal infection Weight APGARs Side of hernia Pre ECMO-Arrest pH Ventilator settings	4374 Neonates with CDH from ELSO registry (2000–2015)
CDH On-ECMO	2018	Pre-ECMO + On-ECMO ECMO settings (pump type) ECMO associated complications (hemorrhage, severe neurologic complication, elevated creatinine, dialysis, tamponade, CPR, sepsis)	4374 Neonates with CDH from ELSO registry (2000–2015)
PIPER	2016	Apgar at 5 minutes <7 Birth weight < 3 kg Age > 10 days CDH MAP <49 mm Hg pO2 < 34 mmHg Patient not on iNO	5455 on VA ECMO, <30 days from ELSO registry (2000–2010)
Neo-RESCUERS	2016	Birth Weight Gestational Age Age Gender Primary Diagnosis Comorbidity Renal Failure pH PaO2/FiO2 iNO	4592 patients, <28 days From ELSO registry (2008–2013)
PED-RESCUERS	2016	Comorbidities Primary diagnosis of Asthma, Bronchiolitis or Pertussis pH PaCO2 Ventilator settings Duration of admission and MV prior to ECMO Milrinone	2458 on ECMO for respiratory failure, 29 days to 18 years from ELSO registry (2009–2014)
P-PREP	2017	Gender Age > 10 Year of ECMO support Primary pulmonary diagnosis Comorbidities PF ratio pH VV vs. VA Mechanical ventilation >14 days HFOV iNO Neuromuscular blockade	4352 patients on ECMO for respiratory failure, >7 days to <18 years from ELSO registry (2001–2013)

ECMONet	2013	PreECMO hospital length of stay Mean Arterial pressure Bilirubin Creatinine Hematocrit	60 adult influenza A patients with respiratory failure from multicenter data (2009 H1N1 Pandemic)
PRESERVE	2013	Age BMI Immunocompromised SOFA>13 MV > 6 days No prone positioning prior to ECMO PEEP <10 Plateau Pressure > 30	140 adult ARDS patients from multicenter data (2008–2012)
RESP	2013	Age Immunocompromised status Mechanical ventilation prior to initiation of ECMO Acute Respiratory Diagnosis CNS dysfunction Acute associated non-pulmonary infection Cardiac Arrest prior to ECMO PaCO2 Neuromuscular blockade prior to ECMO iNO Bicarb. Level Peak inspiratory pressure	2355 adult patients with respiratory failure from ELSO registry (2000–2012)
Roch Score	2014	SOFA score Age Influenza Pneumonia	85 adult patients with ARDS from single center (2009–2013)
VV	2016	Immunocompromised SOFA score Days of MV	116 adult patients with ARDS from single center (2007–2015)
PRESET	2017	Hospital days pre ECMO Mean arterial pressure Lactate pH Platelet	108 adult patients with ARDS from single center (2010–2015)

ECMO = extracorporeal membrane oxygenation, CDH = congenital diaphragmatic hernia, MAP = mean arterial pressure, pO2 = partial pressure of oxygen, iNO = inhaled nitric oxide, VA = veno-arterial, ELSO = Extracorporeal Life Support Organization, CPR = cardiopulmonary resuscitation, PHIS = Pediatric Health Information System, MV = mechanical ventilation, VV = veno-venous, HFOV = high frequency oscillatory ventilation, CNS = central nervous system, iNO = inhaled nitric oxide, BMI = body mass index, bicarb = bicarbonate, SOFA = Sequential Organ Failure Assessment, ICU = intensive care unit, ARDS = acute respiratory distress syndrome, PTSD = post-traumatic stress disorder, HRQL = Health Related Quality of Life.

Table 1.
ECMO mortality prediction scores for respiratory failure.

2.1.3 Pediatric

Two common scores exist to predict mortality in pediatric respiratory failure. The Pediatric Risk Estimation Score for Children Using Extracorporeal Respiratory Support (Ped-RESCUERS) and the newer Pediatric Pulmonary Rescue with Extracorporeal Membrane Oxygenation Prediction (P-PREP) score.

Ped-RESCUERS was developed on patients aged 29 days to 18 years, utilizing the ELSO registry from 2009 to 2014, with the 2013 to 2014 cohort as the validation data set to predict survival to hospital discharge [21]. The model was developed and validated on 2458 pediatric patients undergoing ECMO for respiratory support, with an overall observed mortality rate was 39.8%. In addition to variables of severity of respiratory failure up to 6 hours prior to ECMO initiation (pH and $PaCO_2$), the authors also included the duration of mechanical ventilation and type of mechanical ventilatory support prior to cannulation and specific diagnoses such as pertussis, bronchiolitis and malignancy in the model development (**Table 1**). The model had modest performance with an AUROC of 0.69 in the development cohort and 0.63 in the validation data set. Similar to clinical experience, they found those with bronchiolitis and asthma had relatively better outcomes than those with cancer or pertussis, and those requiring ECMO later in their course had increased mortality. Interestingly higher pre-ECMO $PaCO_2$ was associated with less mortality, the authors speculate this may be due to the association with asthma and bronchiolitis and their subsequent survival benefit [21]. Similar to Neo-RESCUERS, the authors acknowledge the inability to use Ped-RESCUERS as a decision support tool on an individual patient level as the model was only developed on patients already supported on ECMO, but rather as a risk adjustment tool to help facilitate inter-institutional comparisons.

The P-PREP Score was developed and internally validated on 4352 children more than 7 days old to less than 18 years old requiring ECMO for respiratory failure in the ELSO registry between 2008 and 2013 and then externally validated in 2007 patients from the Pediatric Health Information System (PHIS) dataset [22]. Predictive variables included mode of ECMO support, and pre-ECMO variables such as length of mechanical ventilation, severity of hypoxia and diagnosis categories and comorbidities (**Table 1**). As the relative timing of comorbidities to ECMO initiation is not recorded in the ELSO registry, all comorbidities were assumed to be present at the time of ECMO cannulation. Of interest, the year of ECMO support was included in the final P-PREP model given the lower mortality rates in the 2009–2013 era compared to 2001–2009, although not assigned a score in the model calculation. Mode of ECMO support and severity of hypoxia were excluded from the external validation model as these variables are not collected in the PHIS database. The model had modest performance in the development, internal and external validation data sets (AUROC of 0.69, 0.66 and 0.69 respectively). Mortality was significantly higher in patients with two or more extrapulmonary organ system failures. Similar to previous models, P-PREP was limited to patients already supported on ECMO and as such could not be used as a ECMO decision making risk tool but the authors suggest it may aid in prognostication and family counseling for patients supported on ECMO for respiratory failure [22].

2.1.4 Adult

Since the 2009 H1N1 influenza A pandemic, there has been an exponential increase in ECMO use for adult respiratory failure [23] and as such several risk prediction scores have been developed for this population.

Perhaps the earliest widely used score was the ECMOnet score – developed on 60 patients from a multicenter 2009 H1N1 influenza A pandemic cohort [24]. The authors' goal was to add consideration to extrapulmonary organ function, and not just the severity of respiratory failure in risk stratification for VV ECMO use in respiratory failure, aiming to aid in resource allocation and timing of ECMO initiation. Pre-ECMO predictors associated with mortality included hospital length of stay, bilirubin, creatinine, hematocrit and mean arterial pressure with a good model performance with an AUROC of 0.85 (**Table 1**). The results were then validated on an external dataset of 74 patients with acute respiratory distress syndrome (ARDS) supported on ECMO with an AUROC of 0.69. This tool provided early evidence of the importance of the consideration of extrapulmonary organ function at time of ECMO initiation.

The Predicting dEath for Severe ARDS on VV-ECMO (PRESERVE) score was developed on data from 140 patients with refractory ARDS in three French intensive care units from 2008 to 2012 to identify factors associated with death by 6 months post-ICU discharge [25]. A large portion of patients (26%) in this group also had H1N1 influenza. Eight pre-ECMO predictors were identified including age, body mass index, immunocompromised status, prone positioning, sepsis-related organ failure, days of pre-ECMO mechanical ventilation, plateau and positive end expiratory pressures (PEEP) (**Table 1**). Interestingly PF ratio was not found to be associated with mortality, but during enrolment of the development cohort increasing evidence had been mounting on the benefit of prone positioning. When the authors forced it into the model, PF ratio was found to be associated with lower mortality. The PRESERVE model performed well with an AUROC of 0.89 at predicting all cause 6-months post-ICU discharge mortality. The goal of the PRESERVE score was to help clinicians select appropriate candidates, and uniquely they provided details on health-related quality of life (HRQL) evaluation at 6 months, finding high levels of persistent physical and emotional difficulties, including anxiety, depression and post-traumatic stress disorder (PTSD) [24].

The Respiratory Extracorporeal Membrane Oxygenation Survival Prediction (RESP) score is one of the most commonly clinically used and cited scores, developed from the ELSO registry data from 2000 to 2012 to predict survival to hospital discharge [26]. The authors also externally validated the score on the 140 patients used for the development of the PRESERVE score, using commonly available features in both datasets. Diagnostic groups, non-pulmonary infections and central nervous system dysfunction were significant predictors, again highlighting the importance of extrapulmonary organ function prior to ECMO initiation. The RESP score demonstrated the importance of ECMO specific mortality prediction scores as it performed better than simple severity of illness scores such as the simplified acute physiology score (SAPS II) and sequential organ failure assessment (SOFA). The RESP score includes five risk classes, with the lowest and highest classes having 8% and 82% mortality respectively. An important limitation of the score development was inability to incorporate prone positioning, as it was not reported in the ELSO registry data. As with the PRESERVE score, duration of mechanical ventilation above 7 days prior to ECMO initiation was found to be significantly associated with worse outcomes. The authors acknowledge the score limitation in only being developed on patients already supported on ECMO in addition to the lack of detailed biologic data in the ELSO registry beyond the immediate pre-ECMO blood gas values.

Since its development, the RESP score has been further externally validated in several independent studies [27, 28] and studies utilizing external databases comparing both the RESP and PRESERVE score have demonstrated similar accuracy [29, 30]. Though several of their variables overlap, which may explain their similar accuracy (**Table 1**). Interestingly, more recent data has shown that the RESP Score performed poorly at predicting mortality during the Coronavirus disease 2019 (COVID-19) pandemic – with patients in lower risk classes paradoxically having worse survival than those in higher risk classes [31].

The Roch Score was development to identify factors associated with in-hospital mortality in 85 ARDS patients treated with ECMO following referral to an ECMO center between 2009 and 2013 [32]. All patients were cannulated by a mobile ECMO unit prior to transfer to the referral center. ECMO decision making followed criteria with exclusion of patients with prolonged mechanical ventilation or ARDS over 7 days, age above 70 years and those with SOFA scores above 18. The uniqueness of this score's development focusing on referral to an ECMO center, may support its utility in decision to transfer to ECMO centers. It included only limited variables (**Table 1**) including age, SOFA score and influenza diagnosis, making it suitable for timely decisions regarding transfer. The authors identified patients that were under 45 years of age and had a diagnosis of influenza had markedly better prognosis, independent of other organ dysfunctions [32].

Another score is the VV-ECMO mortality score [33], which was developed on a 116 adult patients single center cohort between 2007 and 2015. The authors included only patients with a PF ratio < 70, and independent predictors of in-hospital mortality included pre-ECMO variables such as SOFA score, length of mechanical ventilation and immunocompromised status, which were translated into a simple 3 binary variable predictor. The lowest score had a mortality of 18%, while the highest had a mortality of 88%, and again emphasized the importance of extra-pulmonary organ dysfunction and severity of illness. The authors' goal was to develop a simple risk stratification tool to identify patients with the highest of a poor outcome with VV ECMO, for prognostication or consideration of alternative support modalities if possible.

The PREdiction of Survival on ECMO Therapy Score (PRESET) was derived on 108 ARDS patients between 2010 and 2015 [34]. In this work the authors analyzed the performance of 4 previous mortality risk scores; ECMOnet, RESP, PRESERVE and Roch with only the RESP and ECMOnet score demonstrating good accuracy. There was some evidence that the ECMOnet score was most appropriate only in cohorts of H1N1 patients. The authors then developed a new score, PRESET. The importance of extrapulmonary predictors such as mean arterial blood pressure, lactate, pH, platelets and pre-ECMO hospital length of stay were found. The lowest risk class had a 26% mortality rate, while the highest had a 93% mortality rate. Platelet count prior to ECMO initiation was found to be an important predictor, with a decrease of 100,000/ul associated with 30% increased mortality. These findings were similar to those reported in other critically ill patients [35]. A decrease in pH by 0.1 was also found to increase mortality by 40%. Recent studies have also demonstrated the accuracy of the PRESET score in COVID-19 patients [36].

Some studies have aimed at externally validating several of these scores with varying results, with slightly lower accuracy than initially published in general and with some studies showing superior performance of general severity of illness scores at predicting in-hospital mortality [37–39].

2.2 Cardiac failure

2.2.1 Pediatric

The Pediatric Extracorporeal Membrane Oxygenation Prediction (PEP) model was developed for risk stratifying mortality of all pediatric and neonatal patients requiring ECMO regardless of indication between 2012 and 2014 [40]. The authors included on data from 514 patients from the bleeding and thrombosis on extracorporeal membrane oxygenation (BATE) dataset to predict in-hospital mortality. Variables include indication for ECMO, age, CDH diagnosis, and laboratory markers in the 12 hours prior to ECMO initiation, utilizing the data points most proximal and prior to ECMO for analysis (**Table 2**). As with prior scores developed only on ECMO

Score	Year	Variables	Patient cohort
PEP	2019	Age Indication for ECMO CDH MAS Baseline pH PTT INR Documented blood infection prior to ECMO	514 patients, <19 years, from multicenter data (2012–2014)
Pedi-Save	2022	Age Cardiac diagnostic category Race STAT category pH Acid buffer requirement prior to ECMO Number of cardiac procedures Failure to wean from CPB as ECMO indication	10,091 patients with a cardiac diagnosis, <18 years, from ELSO registry (2001–2015)
SAVE	2015	Age Weight Pre-ECMO organ failure Chronic Renal failure Pre-ECMO cardiac arrest DBP before ECMO >40 mmHg PP before ECMO <20 mmHg Bicarb. <15 mmol/L Duration of intubation prior to initiation of ECMO Peak inspiratory pressure < 20 cmH2O	3846 patients with cardiogenic shock from ELSO registry (2003–2013)
Encourage	2016	Age Sex BMI >25 GCS <6 Creatinine Lactate Prothrombin activity	138 patients with AMI patients from multicenter data (2008–2013)
PREDICT VA-ECMO	2018	On-ECMO pH Lactate Bicarb. Level	205 VA-ECMO from single center (2010–2015)
Simple VA ECMO score	2019	Age Duration of intubation Lactate Platelets Albumin	100 adult patients with cardiogenic shock or cardiac arrest from multicenter data (2010–2017)

Score	Year	Variables	Patient cohort
CASUS	2018	ICU duration Lactate Pressure adjusted heart rate Intubation status Renal function Platelet count Neurologic status	90 adult VA ECMO patients from single center (2011–2012)

ECMO = extracorporeal membrane oxygenation, ELSO = Extracorporeal Life Support Organization, VA = veno-arterial, DBP = diastolic blood pressure, PP = pulse pressure, bicarb = bicarbonate, AMI = acute myocardial infarction, CDH = congenital diaphragmatic hernia, MAS = meconium aspiration syndrome, PTT = partial thromboplastin time, INR = international normalization ratio, STAT = The Society of Thoracic Surgeons-European Association for Cardio-Thoracic Surgery, CPB = cardiopulmonary bypass, PP = pulse pressure, Bicarb = bicarbonate, BMI = body mass index, GCS = Glasgow coma scale.

Table 2.
ECMO mortality prediction scores for cardiac failure.

patients' data, the authors acknowledged the inability to generalize the score for individual patient prediction or selection for ECMO support. The same group then performed an external validation of the PEP score on 4342 patients from the ELSO registry between 2012 and 2014 [41]. They found that the score AUROC decreased from 0.75 on the BATE data to 0.64 on the ELSO data with the most significant decrease in the highest risk deciles.

The Pediatric Survival after Veno-arterial ECMO (Pedi-SAVE) score was recently developed utilizing pediatric cardiac VA-ECMO patients from 2001 to 2015 from the ELSO registry from birth to 18 years of age [42]. The study included 10,091 patients, and both pre- and post-cannulation models were developed. Lowest risk patients in the pre- and post-cannulation groups had a 65% and 74% chance of survival respectively, compared to the highest risk groups having 33% and 22% comparatively. Pre-cannulation factors included type of congenital heart disease with better outcomes in patients with non-single ventricle physiology, age, pH, requirement for acid-buffer administration, number of cardiac procedures, the Society of Thoracic Surgeons-European Association for Cardio-Thoracic Surgery score (STAT), combined cardiopulmonary failure and failure to separate from cardiopulmonary bypass prior to ECMO initiation (**Table 2**). The post-cannulation model included pump flow rates in the first 24 hours on ECMO and on-ECMO complications [42]. The authors concluded that the developed scores could serve in risk adjustment, comparing outcomes between centers and across eras. They also acknowledge the limitations of a registry data-based predictive score with lack of granular patient physiological data, inability to control for data completeness and most importantly the inability to generalize the score to direct individual patient care or guide whether to provide or withdraw ECMO support on the individual patient level.

2.2.2 Adult

Several adult prognostic scores exist for ECMO use in the setting of cardiac failure exist. The survival after veno-arterial ECMO (SAVE) score sought to identify pre-ECMO factors which predict survival to hospital discharge, it utilized 3846 patients from the extracorporeal life support organization registry between 2003 and 2013 [43]. The authors performed further validation on an external dataset of 161 patients who underwent VA ECMO support at a single institution. The developed score included 12 variables including underlying diagnosis leading to cardiogenic shock, age, weight, pre-ECMO organ failure, duration of mechanical ventilation prior to ECMO, pre-ECMO cardiac arrest and hemodynamic profile and degree of metabolic acidosis (**Table 2**). The score gave 5 risk classes with survival percentage ranging from 18 to 75%. On internal validation, the score had an AUROC of 0.68 that increased to 0.9 on external validation. The high accuracy may have been due to the validation set being a participant in the original registry, and it being a high volume highly regimented center. Their findings highlighted the importance of timing for ECMO initiation, with too early use exposing patients to unnecessary complications and too late use proving futile. The SAVE score also outperformed the SOFA score at both cannulation and ICU admission and other ICU severity of illness scores at discriminating patients who did not survive to hospital discharge, once again highlighting the importance of ECMO specific scoring methods [43].

Two other common adult cardiac prognostic scores were developed with more limited populations in mind. The prEdictioN of Cardiogenic shock OUtcome foR AMI (Acute Myocardial Infarction) patients salvaGed by VA-ECMO (ENCOURAGE) score was developed to predict in-ICU mortality from data on 138 patients from 2 ICUs between 2008 and 2013 [44]. Similarly, to the PRESERVE score the authors conducted quality of life assessments on ICU survivors, and found high rates of anxiety, depression and PTSD. Seven pre-ECMO predictive variables were identified (**Table 2**) including age, Glasgow coma score, creatinine, lactate, prothrombin activity, body mass index and sex. The lowest risk group had an 80% survival compared to the highest score group having only a 7% survival. In this group of patients with acute myocardial infraction, the ENCOURAGE score had an AUROC of 0.84 outperforming the SAVE score, and myocardial infraction scores such as the GRACE model [45], Dutch University Hospital Model [46] or the SHOCK Trial and Registry Scoring system [47]. Limitations included that development heavily relied on data from 2 highly specialized and experienced centers, limiting its generalizability, in addition some of the VA ECMO patients having low markers of impaired end organ perfusion (lactate and pH), suggesting either early ECMO initiation or less severe disease at initiation of ECMO.

The PREDICT VA-ECMO score was developed on a single center derivation cohort of 205 all-comers who received VA ECMO from 2010 to 2015, and validated on a cohort from an independent center from 2010 to 2017 [48]. In this work the authors set out to develop a dynamic model to predict hospital survival using on-ECMO variables at multiple time points. Two models were thus developed; the 6-hour PREDICT-VA-ECMO score utilizing variables at 6-hours post ECMO cannulation and the 12-hour PREDICT-VA-ECMO incorporating variables at 1, 6 and 12 hours post cannulation. The PREDICT VA-ECMO score out performed common severity of illness scores, as well as the SAVE score, but with higher accuracy with the 12-hour model compared to the 6-hour model (AUROC of 0.823 and 0.839 respectively), with comparable performance in the external validation cohort. Variables included lactate, pH and bicarbonate (**Table 2**). It demonstrated good prediction accuracy utilizing only a few variables which are easily obtained, and importantly was able to include evaluation of extracorporeal cardiopulmonary resuscitation (eCPR) patients.

Other published scores include a simple scoring system developed on a retrospective cohort of 100 patients between 2010 and 2017 at three institutions, to predict survival to discharge. Five variables were ultimately included, lactate >10 mmol/L, albumin <3 gm/dL and platelets <180,000/uL as well as age and duration of pre-ECMO mechanical ventilation. The lowest score predicted a mortality of 10%, while the highest saw 100% expected mortality [49].

Some studies have also indicated that lactate and urine output are independent predictors of mortality in extracorporeal life support patients, and that the cardiac-surgery score (CASUS) has moderate accuracy compared to simpler severity of illness scores such as SOFA [50].

2.3 Limitations of current approaches

Several limitations exist when evaluating the current landscape of ECMO outcome prediction tools. Although there is good evidence that these scores perform better than standard severity of illness scores, external validation has often shown decreased accuracy. Concerningly many of these scores performed poorly during the novel COVID-19 pandemic, at a time when patient selection and resource allocation was integral [31, 36, 51].

The reasons for poor external validation are likely multifold, while scores developed on large international multicenter registry data should have excellent external validity, this ignores that these databases often have very poor granularity. They fail to account for large center variations which may account for mortality differences [52, 53], including variations in anticoagulation strategies [54], ventilator strategies, timing of ECMO initiation and expertise that may exist in high volume centers [52, 53, 55]. This is especially true when the underlying population receiving ECMO is evolving, as during the COVID-19 pandemic. Static scores lend themselves poorly to changing dynamics in population, as ECMO use has continued to expand since many of these scores have been developed. Furthermore, scores developed utilizing large international registry data and at high volume ECMO centers may translate poorly to centers outside the registry or lower volume or lower resource centers. Particularly concerning is the fact that many of the pediatric and neonatal scores lack any significant external validation, limiting confidence in their deployment.

Another explanation for many of the current generation of ECMO mortality scores' modest performance may be the tendency to rely on accuracy as a measure of performance. Accuracy while made up of sensitivity and specificity, may be less reliable if an outcome of interest is less common. Furthermore, clinicians at the bedside frequently care about positive and negative predictive values, but these are based off prevalence. If centers have large variations in the prevalence of mortality, scores may experience wide variance in their ability to predict the outcome of interest.

Using data from both an institutional database of 15 hospitals in a quaternary referral center and a multinational dataset spanning 42 countries from the COVID-19 pandemic, we evaluated the performance of several ECMO mortality prediction scores; RESP, PRESERVE, Roch and PRESET [56]. In order to more comprehensively evaluate the scores' performance, we reported both accuracy with AUROC and precision with area under the precision recall curve (AUPRC) (**Table 3**). Our results were consistent with previous reports during the pandemic with modest performance of all the studied scores, further emphasizing their limited clinical applicability, especially in the setting of global healthcare system resource limitation.

The current generation of ECMO mortality scores also fails to provide guidance to clinicians in what may be the most vital decision – timing of ECMO initiation. The lack of data regarding the patients' pre-ECMO evolving trajectory and reliance on static variables often immediately prior to ECMO cannulation, in addition to the lack

Dataset		ECMONet	RESP	PRESERVE	Roch	PRESET
Published Datasets	AUROC	0.61	0.64	0.69	0.63	0.66
	AUPRC					
	N	404	601	792	430	388
International dataset	AUROC	0.57	—	—	0.63	0.55
	AUPRC	0.49	—	—	0.71	0.56
	N	328	—	—	214	352
Institutional Dataset	AUROC	0.54	0.53	0.59	0.53	0.61
	AUPRC	0.48	0.49	0.58	0.61	0.61
	N	60	54	21	50	50

AUROC = area under receiver operator curve, AUPRC = area under precision recall curve.

Table 3.
Performance of commonly available ECMO mortality scores in the COVID-19 pandemic.

of a true matched non-ECMO control cohort, significantly limit the utility of all the current scores as clinically applicable decision support tools.

Finally, only two of the scores (ENCOURAGE and PRESERVE) included any data on outcomes aside from mortality, providing information related to quality of life. As mortality improves it likely will become increasingly relevant to begin predicting on meaningful clinical outcomes like neurological function and quality of life.

3. Future directions

The continuously expanding use of ECMO internationally has been coupled by an evolution in biomedical informatics, artificial intelligence and machine learning methodology. This evolution has opened the possibility of exploring more complex machine learning methodologies to develop predictive models to better mirror the clinical decision-making dilemma.

The COVID-19 pandemic has the unmasked the collaborative potential across institutions and even nations to share healthcare data in real time. This opens the possibility to develop more granular multi-institutional databases that expand the currently available registry data. Such databases would open the potential to not only incorporate variables well in advance of ECMO cannulation to better correlate the outcomes with patient trajectories, but also allow the comparison with a propensity matched cohort of non-ECMO critically ill patients to mirror the influence of decision and timing of provision of ECMO support.

The advances in ECMO technology, expanding candidacy and improved outcomes, demonstrate that the use of mortality as an objective outcome has become insufficient. The current landscape of ECMO use mandates a transition from survival to functional neurological outcomes as the goal of predictive modeling. Such an approach requires agreement in the ECMO community on clearly defined definitions for goal neurological outcomes, a task well overdue. Such objective outcomes could then be used as goals in predictive model development to better understand the influence of timing and provision of such high-risk resource-intensive therapy on both individual and system levels.

4. Conclusions

Over the decades since the first deployment of ECMO its application has exponentially increased, and there has been growing interest in developing tools to guide clinical decision making, to help aid in patient selection and prognostication. While several scores have been developed, they share similar limitations secondary to the granularity of the available data, score development approaches, the focus on mortality as the main outcome of interest and reliance on data only from patients supported on ECMO. This has led to continued efforts to refine and a requirement to continuously update these scores. Future directions include a transition from a mortality focused approach to an approach focused on identifying objective short and long-term neurologic outcomes. Additionally, there is a need to develop tools capable of matching the studied ECMO cohort to a non-ECMO cohort of similar severity of illness and then develop tools capable of aiding in both patient selection and determination of the optimal ECMO initiation time to improve both mortality and neurologic outcomes.

Conflict of interest

The authors declare no conflict of interest.

Author details

Neel Shah and Ahmed Said*
Division of Pediatric Critical Care, Department of Pediatrics, Washington University in St. Louis, St. Louis, Missouri, United States of America

*Address all correspondence to: said_a@wustl.edu

References

[1] Hill JD et al. Prolonged extracorporeal oxygenation for acute post-traumatic respiratory failure (shock-lung syndrome). Use of the Bramson membrane lung. The New England Journal of Medicine. 1972;**286**(12):629-634

[2] Bartlett RH et al. Extracorporeal membrane oxygenation (ECMO) cardiopulmonary support in infancy. Trans Am Soc Artif Intern Organs. 1976;**22**:80-93

[3] Peek GJ et al. Efficacy and economic assessment of conventional ventilatory support versus extracorporeal membrane oxygenation for severe adult respiratory failure (CESAR): A multicentre randomised controlled trial. Lancet. 2009;**374**(9698):1351-1363

[4] Krummel TM et al. Alveolar-arterial oxygen gradients versus the neonatal pulmonary insufficiency index for prediction of mortality in ECMO candidates. Journal of Pediatric Surgery. 1984;**19**(4):380-384

[5] Cimma R, Risemberg H, White JJ. A simple objective system for early recognition of overwhelming neonatal respiratory distress. Journal of Pediatric Surgery. 1980;**15**(4):581-585

[6] Dibbins AW, Wiener ES. Mortality from neonatal diaphragmatic hernia. Journal of Pediatric Surgery. 1974;**9**(5):653-662

[7] Shah N, Said AS. Extracorporeal support prognostication-time to move the goal posts? Membranes (Basel). 2021;**11**(7):537-548

[8] Harting M, Davis C, Lally K. Congenital diaphragmatic hernia and ECMO. In: Brogan T, Lequier L, Lorusso R, MacLaren G, Peek G, editors. Extracorporeal Life Support: The ELSO Red Book. 5th ed. Ann Arbor, Michigan: Extracorporeal Life Support Organization; 2017. pp. 133-150

[9] Rafat N, Schaible T. Extracorporeal membrane oxygenation in congenital diaphragmatic hernia. Frontiers in Pediatrics. 2019;**7**:336

[10] Cordier AG et al. Prenatal diagnosis, imaging, and prognosis in congenital diaphragmatic hernia. Seminars in Perinatology. 2020;**44**(1):51163

[11] Schaible T et al. A 20-year experience on neonatal extracorporeal membrane oxygenation in a referral center. Intensive Care Medicine. 2010;**36**(7):1229-1234

[12] McHoney M, Hammond P. Role of ECMO in congenital diaphragmatic hernia. Archives of Disease in Childhood-Fetal and Neonatal Edition. 2018;**103**(2):F178-F181

[13] Puligandla PS et al. Management of congenital diaphragmatic hernia: A systematic review from the APSA outcomes and evidence based practice committee. Journal of Pediatric Surgery. 2015;**50**(11):1958-1970

[14] Bryner BS et al. Congenital diaphragmatic hernia requiring extracorporeal membrane oxygenation: Does timing of repair matter? Journal of Pediatric Surgery. 2009;**44**(6):1165-1172

[15] Tsao K et al. Congenital diaphragmatic hernia in the preterm infant. Surgery. 2010;**148**(2):404-410

[16] Snoek KG et al. Standardized postnatal management of infants with

congenital diaphragmatic hernia in Europe: The CDH EURO consortium consensus-2015 update. Neonatology. 2016;**110**(1):66-74

[17] Sebald M et al. Risk of need for extracorporeal membrane oxygenation support in neonates with congenital diaphragmatic hernia treated with inhaled nitric oxide. Journal of Perinatology. 2004;**24**(3):143-146

[18] Guner YS et al. Development and validation of extracorporeal membrane oxygenation mortality-risk models for congenital diaphragmatic hernia. ASAIO Journal. 2018;**64**(6):785-794

[19] Maul TM, Kuch BA, Wearden PD. Development of risk indices for neonatal respiratory extracorporeal membrane oxygenation. ASAIO Journal. 2016;**62**(5):584-590

[20] Barbaro RP et al. Development and validation of the neonatal risk estimate score for children using extracorporeal respiratory support. The Journal of Pediatrics. 2016;**173**:56-61 e3

[21] Barbaro RP et al. Development and validation of the pediatric risk estimate score for children using extracorporeal respiratory support (Ped-RESCUERS). Intensive Care Medicine. 2016;**42**(5):879-888

[22] Bailly DK et al. Development and validation of a score to predict mortality in children undergoing extracorporeal membrane oxygenation for respiratory failure: Pediatric pulmonary rescue with extracorporeal membrane oxygenation prediction score. Critical Care Medicine. 2017;**45**(1):e58-e66

[23] Organization, E.L.S. ECLS Registry Report. 2022 [cited 2022 June 7 2022]. Available from: https://www.elso.org/Registry/InternationalSummaryandReports/InternationalSummary.aspx

[24] Pappalardo F et al. Predicting mortality risk in patients undergoing venovenous ECMO for ARDS due to influenza a (H1N1) pneumonia: The ECMOnet score. Intensive Care Medicine. 2013;**39**(2):275-281

[25] Schmidt M et al. The PRESERVE mortality risk score and analysis of long-term outcomes after extracorporeal membrane oxygenation for severe acute respiratory distress syndrome. Intensive Care Medicine. 2013;**39**(10):1704-1713

[26] Schmidt M et al. Predicting survival after extracorporeal membrane oxygenation for severe acute respiratory failure. The respiratory extracorporeal membrane oxygenation survival prediction (RESP) score. American Journal of Respiratory and Critical Care Medicine. 2014;**189**(11):1374-1382

[27] Man MY, Shum HP, Lam SM, Yu JSY, King BHS, Yan WW. An external validation of scoring systems in mortality prediction in Veno-venous extracorporeal membrane oxygenation. ASAIO Journal. 2022;**68**(2):255-261

[28] Klinzing S et al. External validation of scores proposed for estimation of survival probability of patients with severe adult respiratory distress syndrome undergoing extracorporeal membrane oxygenation therapy: A retrospective study. Critical Care. 2015;**19**:142

[29] Kang HR et al. A comparative analysis of survival prediction using PRESERVE and RESP scores. The Annals of Thoracic Surgery. 2017;**104**(3):797-803

[30] Brunet J et al. Predicting survival after extracorporeal membrane oxygenation for ARDS:

An external validation of RESP and PRESERVE scores. Respiratory Care. 2017;**62**(7):912-919

[31] Joshi H et al. Respiratory ECMO survival prediction (RESP) score for COVID-19 patients treated with ECMO. ASAIO Journal. 2022;**68**(4):486-491

[32] Roch A et al. Outcome of acute respiratory distress syndrome patients treated with extracorporeal membrane oxygenation and brought to a referral center. Intensive Care Medicine. 2014;**40**(1):74-83

[33] Cheng YT et al. Developing a simple preinterventional score to predict hospital mortality in adult venovenous extracorporeal membrane oxygenation: A pilot study. Medicine (Baltimore). 2016;**95**(30):e4380

[34] Hilder M et al. Comparison of mortality prediction models in acute respiratory distress syndrome undergoing extracorporeal membrane oxygenation and development of a novel prediction score: The PREdiction of survival on ECMO therapy-score (PRESET-score). Critical Care. 2017;**21**(1):301

[35] Thiery-Antier N et al. Is thrombocytopenia an early prognostic marker in septic shock? Critical Care Medicine. 2016;**44**(4):764-772

[36] Tabatabai A et al. Mortality risk assessment in COVID-19 Venovenous extracorporeal membrane oxygenation. The Annals of Thoracic Surgery. 2021;**112**(6):1983-1989

[37] Man M-Y et al. An external validation of scoring Systems in Mortality Prediction in Veno-venous extracorporeal membrane oxygenation. ASAIO Journal. 2022;**68**(2):255-261

[38] Wang R et al. Predictive values of different critical scoring systems for mortality in patients with severe acute respiratory failure supported by extracorporeal membrane oxygenation. Zhonghua Jie He He Hu Xi Za Zhi. 2016;**39**(9):698-703

[39] Maca J et al. Extracorporeal membrane oxygenation survival: External validation of current predictive scoring systems focusing on influenza a etiology. Artificial Organs. 2021;**45**(8):881-892

[40] Bailly DK et al. Development of the pediatric extracorporeal membrane oxygenation prediction model for risk-adjusting mortality. Pediatric Critical Care Medicine. 2019;**20**(5):426-434

[41] Bailly DK et al. External validation of the pediatric extracorporeal membrane oxygenation prediction model for risk adjusting mortality. Perfusion. 2021;**36**(4):407-414

[42] Geisser DL et al. Development of a model for the pediatric survival after Veno-arterial extracorporeal membrane oxygenation score: The Pedi-SAVE score. ASAIO Journal. 2022:9000

[43] Schmidt M et al. Predicting survival after ECMO for refractory cardiogenic shock: The survival after veno-arterial-ECMO (SAVE)-score. European Heart Journal. 2015;**36**(33):2246-2256

[44] Muller G et al. The ENCOURAGE mortality risk score and analysis of long-term outcomes after VA-ECMO for acute myocardial infarction with cardiogenic shock. Intensive Care Medicine. 2016;**42**(3):370-378

[45] Fox KA et al. Management of acute coronary syndromes. Variations in practice and outcome. Findings from the global registry of acute coronary events (GRACE). European Heart Journal. 2002;**23**(15):1177-1189

[46] Cheng JM et al. A simple risk chart for initial risk assessment of 30-day mortality in patients with cardiogenic shock from ST-elevation myocardial infarction. European Heart Journal: Acute Cardiovascular Care. 2016;**5**(2):101-107

[47] Sleeper LA et al. A severity scoring system for risk assessment of patients with cardiogenic shock: A report from the SHOCK trial and registry. American Heart Journal. 2010;**160**(3):443-450

[48] Wengenmayer T et al. Development and validation of a prognostic model for survival in patients treated with venoarterial extracorporeal membrane oxygenation: The PREDICT VA-ECMO score. European Heart Journal: Acute Cardiovascular Care. 2019;**8**(4):350-359

[49] Worku B et al. A simple scoring system to predict survival after Venoarterial extracorporeal membrane oxygenation. The Journal of Extra-Corporeal Technology. 2019;**51**(3):133-139

[50] Hofmann B et al. Cardiac surgery score (CASUS) improves outcome prediction in patients treated with extracorporal life support (ECLS). Perfusion. 2018;**33**(1):36-43

[51] Zayat R et al. Role of extracorporeal membrane oxygenation in critically ill COVID-19 patients and predictors of mortality. Artificial Organs. 2021;**45**(6):E158-E170

[52] Barbaro RP et al. Association of hospital-level volume of extracorporeal membrane oxygenation cases and mortality. Analysis of the extracorporeal life support organization registry. American Journal of Respiratory and Critical Care Medicine. 2015;**191**(8):894-901

[53] Becher PM et al. Procedural volume and outcomes in patients undergoing VA-ECMO support. Critical Care. 2020;**24**(1):291

[54] Seeliger B et al. Comparison of anticoagulation strategies for veno-venous ECMO support in acute respiratory failure. Critical Care. 2021;**24**(1):701

[55] Rabie AA et al. Implementation of new ECMO centers during the COVID-19 pandemic: Experience and results from the Middle East and India. Intensive Care Medicine. 2021;**47**(8):887-895

[56] ISARIC Clinical Characterisation Group, Xue B, Shah N, Yang H, Kannampallil T, Marwali E, et al. 2021 ELSO Meeting Abstracts. ASAIO Journal. 2021;**67**:1-57